AF805326

Anthropometry

Francisco Esparza-Ros ·
Raquel Vaquero-Cristóbal

Anthropometry

Fundamentals of Application and Interpretation

Springer

Francisco Esparza-Ros
International Chair of Kinanthropometry
UCAM Catholic University San Antonio
of Murcia
Murcia, Spain

Raquel Vaquero-Cristóbal
Faculty of Sport Sciences
University of Murcia
Murcia, Spain

ISBN 978-3-031-77534-5 ISBN 978-3-031-77535-2 (eBook)
https://doi.org/10.1007/978-3-031-77535-2

The original submitted manuscript has been translated into English. The translation was done using artificial intelligence. A subsequent revision was performed by the author(s) to further refine the work and to ensure that the translation is appropriate concerning content and scientific correctness. It may, however, read stylistically different from a conventional translation.

Translation from the Spanish language edition: "Antropometría: Fundamentos para la aplicación e interpretación" by Francisco Esparza-Ros and Raquel Vaquero-Cristóbal, © Francisco Esparza-Ros y Raquel Vaquero-Cristóbal 2023. Published by Editorial Aula Magna. All Rights Reserved.

© The Editor(s) (if applicable) and The Author(s), under exclusive license to Springer Nature Switzerland AG 2025

This work is subject to copyright. All rights are solely and exclusively licensed by the Publisher, whether the whole or part of the material is concerned, specifically the rights of reprinting, reuse of illustrations, recitation, broadcasting, reproduction on microfilms or in any other physical way, and transmission or information storage and retrieval, electronic adaptation, computer software, or by similar or dissimilar methodology now known or hereafter developed.
The use of general descriptive names, registered names, trademarks, service marks, etc. in this publication does not imply, even in the absence of a specific statement, that such names are exempt from the relevant protective laws and regulations and therefore free for general use.
The publisher, the authors and the editors are safe to assume that the advice and information in this book are believed to be true and accurate at the date of publication. Neither the publisher nor the authors or the editors give a warranty, expressed or implied, with respect to the material contained herein or for any errors or omissions that may have been made. The publisher remains neutral with regard to jurisdictional claims in published maps and institutional affiliations.

Cover image: Kirill Gorlov/stock.adobe.com

This Springer imprint is published by the registered company Springer Nature Switzerland AG
The registered company address is: Gewerbestrasse 11, 6330 Cham, Switzerland

If disposing of this product, please recycle the paper.

Foreword

It is my privilege to write the foreword to this overdue text on Anthropometry, its theory and its applications. It is written by an internationally-recognized orthopaedic surgeon and anthropometrist and his no-less-able young colleague—already well-recognized as a practitioner and publisher in sports science and anthopometry in her own right.

There has been a small number of comprehensive teaching texts on the practice and theory of Anthropometry in the last thirty years, most of which need updating in the light of new knowledge. This book achieves that.

A glance at the Table of Contents reveals a comprehensive coverage of key areas which aspiring anthropometrists need to be very familiar with. Of particular value are those chapters on analysis and application which ably bridge the gap between theory and practice, a bridging that is so necessary to achieve competence and purpose.

I recommend this book to you and look forward to its recognition as a valuable addition to the arsenal of all those involved in the key endeavour of better understanding the structure and function of the human body.

Upper Hutt, New Zealand
June 2024

Prof. Mike Marfell-Jones

Acknowledgements

To Mario Albaladejo-Saura, Adrián Mateo-Orcajada, Alejandro Espeso-García and Tomás Abelleira-Lamela for their invaluable help in the development of this book.

Synopsis

The science of Anthropometry is gaining an increasing number of followers, as it allows for a valid, reliable and cheap assessment of body composition and other interesting variables from the point of view of health and sport. However, not many books have addressed the anthropometric technique from its foundations. This book deals with issues to consider during an anthropometric assessment, such as the physical approach to the subject during the anthropometric assessment, or the factors to consider so that the data obtained are valid and reliable. It also clearly and concisely addresses the approach to body composition with anthropometry, what somatotype is, and how it is interpreted, and how anthropometry can be used to obtain proportionality values, which are very useful for the detection of sporting talents. Finally, the application of anthropometry in two of the fields where anthropometry is most used: the field of sport from the basics to elite sport, and health. All of this is conducted under the perspective of two of the world's leading experts in kinanthropometry, with the goal for the reader to acquire knowledge on every aspect of anthropometry, from the basics to in-depth knowledge of this science.

Contents

About the Authors

Francisco Esparza-Ros born on November 27th, 1957 in Murcia (Spain), he graduated in Medicine and Surgery in 1981 from the University of Murcia. He is a medical specialist in Sports Traumatology and also in Physical Education and Sports Medicine. In 1996 he obtained the title of Doctor in Medicine and Surgery from the University of Valencia, with a "cum laude" distinction, and since 1997 he has been a professor at the Catholic University San Antonio de Murcia, where he has been leading the Master's in Sports Traumatology since 2010 and has been the director of the International Chair of Kinanthropometry since 2015. His experience with anthropometry began in 1987, being the author of numerous scientific documents related to this discipline. He holds the title of Level 4 criterion anthropometrist from the International Society for the Advancement in Kinanthropometry (ISAK). He has been the General Secretary of the ISAK for 10 years and Vice President of the ISAK for 6 years. Currently, he is the President of this Society, being the first Spanish speaker to hold this position.

Raquel Vaquero-Cristóbal born on April 12th, 1989 in Valladolid (Spain), she graduated in Physical Activity and Sports Sciences in 2011 from the University of Murcia (UMU), receiving an Extraordinary Award and End of University Education Mention. She completed her doctorate in 2017 within the programme of Physical Activity and Sports Sciences at the Catholic University San Antonio de Murcia (UCAM), with a cum laude distinction. She worked as a professor and researcher at the Faculty of Sport at the UCAM from 2017 to 2023. Since then, she has been working as a professor and researcher at the Faculty of Sports Sciences at the UMU. She has extensive experience in teaching anthropometry to students from different disciplines. She is a Level 4 criterion anthropometrist from the International Society for the Advancement in Kinanthropometry (ISAK) and has been a member of the Executive Committee of this Society from 2018 to the present. In addition, she is currently the General Secretary of the ISAK. During her research career, she has published various books and scientific articles related to kinanthropometry. She is one of the creators of the ISAK Metry software for anthropometric assessment.

History of Anthropometry and Evolution of the International Society for the Advancement of Kinanthropometry (ISAK)

1

Abstract

The present chapter is an introduction to anthropometry as a science. It describes a terminological approach to this concept and specifies that it is based on the measurement of various dimensions of the human body, from basic measurements to skinfolds, girths, lengths and heights, and breadths and depths, using specialised scientific techniques. It explains that the International Society for the Advancement of Kinanthropometry (ISAK) standardises the measurement protocol of these variables, offering certification courses for anthropometrists, and it details the structure and operation of the ISAK accreditation system. The evolution of anthropometry throughout history is also specified, covering the main milestones in relation to this discipline; as well as the evolution of the standardisation of the anthropometric technique, which culminates in the publication of the "International Protocol for Anthropometric Assessment" by ISAK, ensuring uniformity in measurements worldwide

Keywords

Anthropometry • ISAK • Standardisation • History • Accreditation • Protocol • Measurements

1.1 Introduction to Anthropometry

The International Society for the Advancement of Kinanthropometry (ISAK) was founded as an organization of individuals whose scientific and professional work is related to anthropometry.

Anthropometry is composed of two terms, ánthropos (man) and metrya (measure). Anthropometry refers to the procedures and scientific processes that allow obtaining both superficial anatomical dimensional measurements, such as basic measurements, skinfolds, girths, lengths and heights, and breadths and depths

© The Author(s), under exclusive license to Springer Nature Switzerland AG 2025
F. Esparza-Ros and R. Vaquero-Cristóbal, *Anthropometry*,
https://doi.org/10.1007/978-3-031-77535-2_1

in the human body, through specialized equipment. Another possible definition would be the one that defines it as the science that deals with the comparative measurements of the human body, its different parts, and their proportions.

Kinanthropometry refers to the measurement of man in motion, not movement in terms of moving, not only to the development of the human being (from child to adult, and from adult to elderly person), but also to the dependent changes that conditional variables such as nutritional habits and physical exercise exert on the individual.

Therefore, anthropometry refers to the measurements made, while kinanthropometry uses these measurements to establish relationships with other aspects such as movement/physical activity, development or physiology. However, for a matter of homogenization of the nomenclature, anthropometry will be used throughout the document. Therefore, it is a science that studies the relationship between human structure and function (Ross et al., 1978). In addition, it is the academic discipline that is based on the use of anthropometric measurements in relation to other scientific parameters and/or thematic areas such as human movement, physiology or applied health sciences. This allows studying the morphology (the shape of the individual), the body composition, and the proportion of the human body through the use of measurements, which allows us to know and better understand movement, in relation to the activity of human beings (exercise, development, growth, nutrition, or health).

For this, ISAK has taken care of standardizing the measurement process, protocolising the anatomical points, the measurement techniques, and the anthropometric material used. For this purpose, it includes Level 3 (instructor) and Level 4 (criterion) instructors, who are the ones who teach Level 1 (restricted profile) or Level 2 (complete profile) courses. In this way, students who successfully complete the ISAK training courses obtain a certification, recognized in the scientific field, indicating that they are accredited to take high-quality measurements.

1.2 Background. Origins and History

Throughout history, there have been numerous representations among ancient cultures that mention some kind of relationship with kinanthropometry, and are considered as prior events to highlight in the history of this discipline. Thus, between the years 450–430 BC, the Doryphoros of Polykleitos represented the ideal model of shapes and proportions, which could be considered the first "reference human", using a head as a reference measurement to measure the stretch stature of individuals. During the Renaissance, art and science became very important, and it was during this time that advances were made on knowledge of symmetry and proportion, and between the years 1400 and 1600, reference scientists such as Leone Battista Alberti, Albrecht Dürer, Leonardo da Vinci, Michelangelo or Galileo Galilei, as well as the anatomical drawings of Andreas Vesalius, all contributed to shaping the basis of anthropometry.

Another important author is Adolphe Quetelet (1796–1874), who observed certain constant patterns in the behaviour of certain data from anthropometric variables, which led him to perform an analysis with applied mathematical techniques, giving rise to the body mass index.

In the nineteenth century, anthropologists and palaeontologists began to use engineering tools to measure the fossils of species that lived in other eras, among which were human bones. Later in this same century, biostatistics emerged, which allowed anthropometry to be linked to function, thanks to a series of mathematical works that allowed correlations to be found to discover the measurements and different values of an individual.

Already in the twentieth century, Howard V. Meredith, in the United States, made a great contribution to anthropometry, facilitating the development of anthropometry as a tool for studying the health of populations. During the 1940s, William Sheldon created the somatotype as a description of the physique summarised into three aspects: adiposity, musculoskeletal robustness, and slimness, associating these aspects with the psychological variables and personality traits of the subjects.

In 1942, Albert Behnke, a military man in charge of rescuing some submariners, contributed great amount of knowledge on body composition, as he had to perform the necessary calculations on the body composition of the soldiers who were inside the submarine in order to evacuate them. For this, he generated some regression equations for skinfolds as a method for estimating the body composition of the submariners.

During the 1960s, Barbara Heath and Lindsay Carter corrected and modified the original somatotype designed by William Sheldon (1940s), generating an objective estimation system from anthropometric measurements. This is the somatotype that is currently used, which has great relevance in the study of anthropometry.

Later, in 1968, Carter led an anthropometric measurement project at the Mexico Olympic Games (OG), with this event being of special relevance to the field of anthropometry, just as the Montreal Olympic Games Anthropological Project (MOGAP) carried out at the 1976 OG in Montreal. Both moments are key to the history of anthropometry, as it was introduced into the field of sport, specifically in the OG.

In 1976, Jim Tanner, at the Institute of Child Health in England, began his Harpenden longitudinal study of growth and development, of great international relevance, designing, together with his collaborators, the skinfold caliper, which bears the same name as the project (Harpenden), and which is currently considered one of the best skinfold calipers.

Finally, one of the most relevant events for anthropometry, also considered a turning point, is the study of corpses carried out in Brussels in the early 70s and 80s (1971–1983) by Alan Martin, Donald T. Drinkwater, and Jan Clarys, among others, in which 25 corpses of 12 men and 13 women were included. This changed the course of anthropometry, providing one of the greatest advances in this science, thanks to contributions to the different regression equations that have emerged from this study, allowing for a more precise estimation of body composition.

The 90s brought major advances in diagnostic imaging technology, especially with the arrival of bone densitometry (DEXA), computed axial tomography (CAT) and nuclear magnetic resonance (NMR), with these methods being primarily used to estimate bone mineral density, visceral adiposity of the abdominal region, and more recently, muscle mass. These methods have a good correlation index with anthropometric indicators that are related to pathologies associated with excess visceral fat.

1.3 History and Evolution of ISAK

Following the cadaver study of 1983, ISAK was born in Glasgow on July 20th, 1986, with the purpose of creating and maintaining an international network of professionals representing the global community that transcends geography, politics and the boundaries of different disciplines, in order to establish a dynamic area of scientific work. Prior to its foundation, the International Working Group on Kinanthropometry (IWGK) had been created in 1978 under the auspices of the ICSSPE (International Council of Sport Science and Physical Education), a council in turn associated with the UNESCO. ISAK has also received Bureau Veritas certification (ISO 9001) since 2015, which accredits the quality of compliance with ISAK's internal regulations established in the Handbook, and transparency in the work carried out by ISAK's General Secretariat in managing ISAK courses, certifying its credibility.

1.4 Structure of ISAK

ISAK is governed by an executive committee composed of five officers (the president, the vice-president, the secretary-general, the treasurer, and the past-president) and up to five members. The current composition of the ISAK Council can be found on its website (www.isak.global). On the same website, the history of presidents and general secretaries of the Society can also be found.

1.5 Growth and Development of ISAK

The ISAK has a website (www.isak.global) where those interested can find information about its history, committee and courses, among other aspects. This website is a great advancement for the ISAK, as it allows one to check the membership status of each member, informing about whether an anthropometrist is up to date, and their accreditation remains valid. In addition to this, one can search for ISAK-approved courses by city, country, level, etc.

In addition, ISAK has a tool, called ISAK Metry, which all members of the Society can access for free. This tool allows for the annotation of subject measurements, after which it can automatically generate anthropometric reports, being able to make comparisons between these reports based on four different profiles: (1) express profile, for the evaluation of plastic components; (2) restricted profile (21 measurements of the ISAK restricted profile); (3) 5-component profile, with the necessary measurements for the calculation of body composition with Kerr's 5-component model; and (4) complete profile, which includes the 43 measurements of the complete profile described by the ISAK.

1.6 ISAK Biennial Congress

Every two years, the biennial congress of the ISAK takes place, which is the meeting point for ISAK members where the scientific advances developed by the different research groups are presented. You can find a list on the Society's website: www.isak.global.

1.7 Standardisation of Anthropometric Technique

The first point of reference in the process of standardising anthropometric techniques is found in the Frankfurt agreement of 1880. This is the first record of an attempt to standardise these processes. Subsequently, in the years 1902 and 1912 in Monaco and Geneva, respectively, congresses were held in which the techniques for measuring 49 anthropometric variables were described.

In the 1960s, in the International Biological Program (IBP), driven by England, the left side was established as the reference for taking measurements, unlike the American measurers who established the right side. In 1988, the Arlie conference took place in Virginia (USA), in which Lohman, Roche, and Matorrell, exponents of American techniques, published the Anthropometric Standardisation Reference Manual, this being a document that has especially been the reference for American measurers.

During this standardisation process, the standards and measurements laboratory of the Australian Institute of Sport decided to standardise the technique and knowledge of anthropometry as part of the national health and sports project.

Finally, a turning point in this evolution of the standardisation of anthropometric techniques is the publication of the book Anthropometric in 1996, which was later corrected and improved in the publication of the ISAK International Standards for Anthropometric Assessment in 2001, and subsequently updated in 2006, 2011, and 2019, with the latter being the current version.

This leads to the manual called "International Protocol for Anthropometric Assessment" being a useful and reference tool for measuring the restricted profile and full profile, while also used by all anthropometrists with the aim that different measurements are not made in different parts of the world.

This manual contains guidelines and procedures on techniques for correctly performing anthropometric measurements. It is essential to follow the appropriate protocol to perform the measurements in the same anatomical place and with the same anthropometric technique, taking into account that the instruments used for the measurements must be carefully selected for correct measurement.

1.8 Anthropometric Studies Carried Out in Olympic Games, International Championships and Big Data in Athlete Studies

To date, seven studies have been carried out in different Olympic Games, international championships and big data in athlete studies:

- Olympic Games Mexico 1968. Anthropometric profiles at the Mexico Olympic Games of the Olympic athletes in Mexico City. Led by Carter along with Hebbelinck and Garay.
- Olympic Games Montreal 1976. The MOGAP, the anthropometric project at the Montreal Olympic Games, was developed with Carter, Hebbelinck, Lavieere, Ross, Malina, Bouchard, Yuhasz and Borms, the latter being the first president of the ISAK.
- World Swimming Championships Perth, 1991. 6th world championship of the International Swimming Federation (FINA) in Perth (Australia). Anthropometry project in water sports. With Carter along with Ackland, Mazza, Ross, Marfell-Jones and Porta.
- Olympic Games Sydney 2000. Anthropometry project of rowing, canoe and Olympic kayak with Ackland, Kerr, Hume, Ross, Ong, Ridge and Broad.
- 2002 Oceania Weightlifting Championship, New Zealand. With Keogh, Hume, Pearson, Mellow and Sheerin.
- River Plate Football Club (Buenos Aires), 2008. Extensive study by Francis Holway.
- Malaysia Badminton World Championships, 2008. Carried out with Zakaria, Ali, Razali, Hume, Png and Aziz.

It should be noted that the last study carried out with elite athletes is from many years ago, because in this field, athletes are often reluctant to be evaluated before the competition, and much less during the competition, with this being a great difficulty to consider for the study of this population of athletes.

1.9 ISAK Accreditation System

During this standardisation process, the Australian Institute of Sport, under the responsibility of Dr. Chris Gore and with the help of Deborah Kerr, generated the four-level accreditation scheme currently known (Level 1–4). Subsequently, the programme approved by the ISAK is known as the International Accreditation Programme in Kinanthropometry (IAAS). In 1996, mechanisms for certification in anthropometry were established, using the Australian method, and the proposed method was evaluated four years later (Brisbane, 2000). In 2002, in Manchester, this method was reviewed and finally approved in Thessaloniki in 2004.

This method has led to four levels of accreditation:

- Level 1: technicians, restricted profile. The anthropometrist is trained in taking 21 measurements, which include 4 basic measurements, 8 skinfolds, 6 girths and 3 breadths. This level 1 is more than sufficient for the assessment of plastic components (adiposity and muscle), which is what the professional usually requires on a daily basis. This level is usually obtained by graduates in sports science, nutrition, or health sciences. The information obtained with these 21 measurements allows for the monitoring of health variables, growth and the calculation of the somatotype, body composition, and basic issues of proportionality. It provides a basic theoretical understanding of the applications of anthropometry.
- Level 2: technicians, full profile. The anthropometrist is trained in taking 43 measurements, which include 4 basic measurements, 8 skinfolds, 13 girths, 9 lengths and heights, and 9 breadths and depths. It offers a more complete range of measurements and is therefore intended for people who want to delve into anthropometry, either because they need to conduct research in specific studies, they need information on structural components (bone structure), or they want to approach body composition from Kerr's 5-component model. It provides, in addition, a greater understanding and interpretation of the theoretical concepts of anthropometry.
- Level 3: instructor. The anthropometrist is trained in theoretical, pedagogical and practical content so that they can teach ISAK courses. Thus, Level 3 will be obtained after passing the accredited course for the training and accreditation of level 1 and 2 anthropometrists. It requires an adequate precision in the 43 anthropometric measurements and possesses sufficient theoretical and practical knowledge. With a level 3 accreditation, what is sought is to make good teachers, being much more intense both in preparation and in face-to-face load than the previous ones.
- Level 4: criterion anthropometrist. It involves the responsibility of training and examining level 3 anthropometrists, as well as the right to teach and examine the other two levels. The acquisition of this Level 4 involves a series of requirements underlining a long experience and contribution in ISAK, a high level of theoretical knowledge, participation in the teaching and instruction of ISAK courses, publications or contributions related to large anthropometric projects. Once the criteria are met, accreditation to Level 4 is proposed, with an anonymous committee making the decision to grant such accreditation.

The list of level 4s with valid certification can be found on the ISAK website: www.isak.global.

Finally, it should be noted that the validity of the certification is four years and four months for level 1, and four years and six months for levels 2, 3 and

4, so re-certification will be required after this time, regardless of the level of the anthropometrist, which allows certifying that the quality and validity of the measurement continues to be adequate.

1.10 Questionnaire

1. The term "anthropometry" refers to:
   (a) Procedures and scientific processes that allow obtaining surface anatomical measurements in the human body through specialised material.
   (b) The science that deals with comparative measurements of the human body, its different parts and their proportions.
   (c) The academic discipline that allows studying the morphology, body composition and proportion of the human body with measurements, which allows better understanding and comprehension of movement, in relation to human activity.
   (d) All of the above are true.
2. The standardisation of the anthropometric measurement process has been carried out by:
   (a) The World Health Organisation (WHO).
   (b) The International Olympic Committee (IOC).
   (c) The International Society for the Advancement of Kinanthropometry (ISAK).
   (d) There is no standardisation for anthropometric measurements.
3. In relation to the origins and history of anthropometry:
   (a) There are not many representations of the use of anthropometry in history.
   (b) Its origin is exclusively linked to the scientific field.
   (c) During the twentieth century, significant advances and contributions were made to anthropometry.
   (d) The studies carried out on cadavers by Martin, Drinkwater and Clarys are not particularly relevant.
4. Indicate the false statement regarding the history of the ISAK:
   (a) Until the creation of the ISAK, there had been no association dedicated to the study of anthropometry.
   (b) The ISAK was created in Glasgow in 1986.
   (c) The purpose of ISAK is to create and maintain an international network of professionals in order to establish a dynamic area of scientific work around this discipline.
   (d) The ISAK has current accreditations that guarantee its credibility at an international level.
5. Regarding kinanthropometry:
   (a) The twenty-first century has brought about significant advances in diagnostic imaging technology, leading to new methods with which to analyse body composition.

   (b) The ISAK organises a biennial congress, in different places around the world.
   (c) The undertaking of macro-studies in large sports competitions is an active line within kinanthropometry.
   (d) All of the above are true.
6. The executive board of the ISAK is composed of:
   (a) Up to 3 members (president, secretary and member).
   (b) Up to 6 members (president, vice-president and four members).
   (c) Up to 4 members (president, vice-president, secretary and member).
   (d) Up to five official members and five members.
7. Regarding the standardisation of anthropometric measurements throughout history, indicate the false statement:
   (a) Since the nineteenth century, there has been a common standardisation across all countries regarding the anthropometric method.
   (b) In the International Biological Program driven by England, the measurement on the left side of the body was established, unlike what was established by American authors.
   (c) Between 1902 and 1912, at the Monaco and Geneva congresses respectively, measurement techniques for 49 anthropometric variables were described.
   (d) The ISAK, based on the book Anthropometrica (1996), published the ISAK International Standards for Anthropometric Assessment in 2001, which has been revised on several occasions.
8. Indicate the correct statement regarding the ISAK Metry:
   (a) The ISAK Metry is a tool developed by the ISAK and available to all its members.
   (b) This tool allows you to annotate and generate reports for data interpretation.
   (c) The ISAK Metry has different profiles with different variables depending on the user's interest.
   (d) All of the above are correct.
9. Regarding the major studies conducted in anthropometry, indicate the true answer:
   (a) There are updated anthropometric studies conducted with a large number of elite athletes.
   (b) To date, seven major studies have been conducted at the Olympic Games, international championships and big data in elite athletes.
   (c) In general, elite athletes are willing to undergo anthropometric assessments around competitive periods.
   (d) All of the above are true.
10. Regarding the ISAK accreditation system, indicate the false answer:
   (a) The ISAK accreditation system is based on four levels.
   (b) Level 1 refers to technicians, restricted profile; level 2 refers to technicians, full profile; level 3 refers to instructors; level 4 refers to criterion anthropometrists.

(c) According to the accreditation system, it is not necessary to meet any requirement to access the training of the different accreditation levels.
(d) Once a training course has been completed, the certification is valid for four years and four months for level 1, and four years and six months for levels 2, 3 and 4.

Answers:
1d, 2c, 3c, 4a, 5b, 6d, 7a, 8d, 9b, 10c.

Bibliography

Carter, J. E. L. (1982). *Physical structure of Olympic athletes Part I: The Montreal Olympic games anthropological project*. Karger.

Carter, J. E. L., & Heath, B. H. (1990). *Somatotyping: Development and application*. Cambridge University Press.

Esparza F. (1993). *Manual of kinanthropometry*. FEMEDE.

Esparza-Ros, F., & Vaquero-Cristóbal, R. (2021). Evolution of kinanthropometry at an international level and in Spain. In J. E. Sirvent & J. R. Alvero (Eds.), *Kinanthropometry and its applications* (pp. 11–26). Universitat D'Alacant.

Esparza-Ros, F., Vaquero-Cristóbal, R., & Marfell-Jones, M. (2019). *International protocol for anthropometric assessment*. International Society for the Advancement of Kinanthropometry.

Norton, K., & Olds, T. (1996). *Anthropometric*. New South Wales Press.

Ross, W. D., Hebbelinck, M., Brown, S. R., & Faulkner, R. A. (1978). Kinanthropometric landmarks and terminology. In R. J. Shepard & H. Lavalle (Eds.), *Physical fitness assessment* (pp. 44–50). Charles C. Thomas Publishers.

Ross, W. D., Hebbelinck, M., Van Gheluwe, B., & Lemmens, M. L. (1972). Kinanthropométrie et l'Apretiation de l'Erreur de Mesure. *Kinanthropologie, 4*, 23–24.

Ethics and Proxemics

2

Abstract

This chapter addresses the importance of ethics and proxemics in anthropometry, focusing on respect and consideration for individuals who are being evaluated. It begins by explaining what proxemics is, that is, the classification of interpersonal distances and their effect on interpersonal behaviour. The importance of respecting personal space during anthropometric measurements is highlighted. Next, the ethical considerations to bear in mind when performing anthropometric measurements are detailed. This includes respecting the dignity, diversity, and rights of individuals, as well as avoiding any type of physical or emotional harm during the measurements. Ethical and legal recommendations are offered, such as obtaining informed consent before performing measurements and ensuring that established ethical principles are followed. The requirements for the subjects to be measured are detailed, including appropriate clothing, skin care, and other considerations related to the comfort and privacy of the individual. In addition, recommendations for measurers when performing anthropometric measurements are presented, as well as issues to consider regarding language. The importance of adapting measurement techniques to ensure the safety and well-being of the evaluated individual is emphasised, always prioritising respect and ethics in all interactions.

Keywords

Proxemics • Ethics • Spatial distances • Informed consent • Privacy • Well-being • Care

© The Author(s), under exclusive license to Springer Nature Switzerland AG 2025

F. Esparza-Ros and R. Vaquero-Cristóbal, *Anthropometry*,
https://doi.org/10.1007/978-3-031-77535-2_2

2.1 Introduction

Ethics and proxemics may be a priori unknown topics, but they are very important issues within anthropometry as it deals with human beings, aside from the close physical proximity needed when taking measurements. They must be respected, and for this, different aspects that are discussed below need to be considered.

2.2 What Is Proxemics?

Proxemics derives from the term "proximus", which comes from Latin, and means next or close. This concept is defined as the study of spatial distances between people and their effect on interpersonal behaviour. Thus, proxemics is a term that deals with the spatial closeness between people. It could be said that proxemics is the response and attitude of a human being to a situation of closeness and proximity with another person, and this, as is logical, will depend on the existing relationship between the individuals. Thus, the way of responding to the proximity of another person, will be different depending on whether it is a relative, a friend or a teacher, for example. Also influencing this closeness, in the first place, is the physical distance between two individuals. Thus, the reaction is different if the "vital space" is invaded by being too close, for example, inside a lift; or if one stays far away and is distant.

The concept of proxemics was used by anthropologist Edward Hall in 1963, when discussing people's reactions depending on the distance between them, quantifying it. He was the first scientist who created a field that currently establishes that:

- *Intimate distance*: when the interpersonal separation is between 15 and 45 cm.
- *Personal distance*: when interpersonal separation is between 46 and 120 cm.
- *Social distance*: when interpersonal separation is between 120 and 360 cm.
- *Public distance*: when the interpersonal separation is above 360 cm.

It should be noted that with the measurement techniques of anthropometry, the personal space of the subject to be measured is invaded, regularly entering the realm of personal distance, to which we must add that there is physical contact, so respect for the subject to be measured must be paramount. In this sense, one must know how to measure and do it correctly, as without the correct handling of the distance, very uncomfortable situations will be caused for the person who is being measured.

2.3 Ethical Considerations

Ethical behaviour has been defined as honesty, fairness, and equity, in interpersonal, professional, and academic relationships, and in research activities to which everyone should adjust (Hollings & Hume, 2018). Ethical behaviour respects the dignity, diversity, and rights of individuals and groups of people.

The anthropometrist, when preparing to take a measurement, must be aware that there are some ethical considerations that may vary depending on personal factors of the subjects to be assessed, the measurements that are intended to be taken, and the place where it is intended to be performed. Thus, it may be necessary to pay special attention to ethical behaviour when assessing people of the opposite sex, of a different ethnicity or culture, who present a functional diversity, or who are not familiar with anthropometric measurements. On the other hand, consideration should be given to whether the measurements that are intended to be taken are appropriate and possible, always avoiding any kind of harm, whether physical or emotional to the person being assessed. Regarding the space where the measurements are to be taken, it is most advisable to have a sufficiently large, private, and quiet place, where the anthropometric assessment can be carried out without the person feeling uncomfortable. In addition to these ethical considerations, the anthropometrist should adopt a responsible behaviour regarding their professional work, striving to maintain objectivity and integrity at all times and respecting the subjects and their cultural environment.

2.4 Recommendations from an Ethical and Legal Point of View

The usefulness and information provided by an anthropometric assessment can be observed from different contexts. In this sense, from a scientific point of view, before carrying out an anthropometric assessment, all measurement procedures used for the research must be approved by the ethics committee of the corresponding institution, with the anthropometrists also ensuring that the principles approved in the Helsinki declaration and the Code of the World Medical Association are respected at all times.

In addition, when the subject goes to an anthropometric service, the first step is to explain how the assessment will proceed, what kind of study is going to be carried out, and in what way, as ignorance of the procedures can cause insecurity in the person who is going to be assessed. In fact, it is advisable to send this information before the measurement, so that the subject comes prepared for it. Also, it is advisable to show the measurement techniques through a video, so that they obtain first-hand knowledge about the procedure to be followed.

Next, the informed consent document will be presented, a document through which the individual confirms that they are aware of everything that will occur in the procedure, and thereby confirms in writing that they are willing to participate in the measurement. At this time, in addition to providing them with the information in writing, the protocol should be explained verbally. It should be clarified that they can withdraw from the measurements at any time if they feel uncomfortable, without needing to provide a reason and without any prejudice to the subject. An explanation about the treatment of the data should also be provided, by specifying that no personal data will be published in any case, and the contact information of the person responsible for this data should also be provided. It is important that the person who will be assessed signs the document before starting, or in the case of being a minor or a subject unable to communicate a conscious decision, the informed consent must be read and signed by their father, mother or legal guardian.

It is highly recommended that the measurements be carried out in the presence of witnesses, and this is especially important in the case of minors.

2.5 Requirements for the Subjects

1. *Subject's type of clothing.* It is recommended that men wear tight shorts, and women wear tight shorts and a sports top. The sports top should not be too loose so as not to hinder marking certain points, especially the subscapular and subscapular skinfold. Alternatively, a bikini or swimsuit can be worn. It is advisable to send the subject an example of clothing in advance so they know how to present themselves for the measurements. In any case, the anthropometric assessment should be avoided with the subject in underwear and with the torso bare in the case of women.
2. *Skin care.* The subject should be reminded before each assessment to come without creams or oils applied to the skin, as this would make measurement difficult. The anthropometrist should palpate carefully, without being aggressive so as not to cause bruises, and firmly at the same time but without harming the subject.

2.6 Recommendations for the Measurer

1. *Punctuality and organisation.* Temporal organisation should be a key aspect, so the subjects are not kept waiting, making the measurement more comfortable.
2. *Haptics.* This refers to the sociocultural aspects of touch. In anthropometric measurements, it is inevitable to touch the person in certain measurements, so one must be aware of how this can affect the person depending on their sociocultural context and take the necessary measures to reduce any discomfort that may occur.
3. *Modesty.* When a subject proceeds to undress, situations where they are looked at directly should be avoided. The measurer will avoid being in front while the subject undresses, and will indicate a place where they can change.
4. *Ticklishness.* When a subject is ticklish, it is advisable to do it quickly but correctly, get there fast, grab and take the skinfold.

5. *Dermographism.* This is known as "writing on the skin". It appears in some patients/athletes, who after the measurements may present a skin reaction to being touched, with redness and skin irritation. In this situation, special caution should be taken as temporary marks can be generated, which may be uncomfortable for the patient. It is usually a benign process and the skin reaction disappears after a few hours. In the case of any type of lesion, the use of gloves will be necessary.
6. *Nails.* The anthropometrist's nails should be at an intermediate length, as long nails do not allow for good measurements, but if they are excessively short they do not allow for guide marks on the skin, which are very useful for locating anatomical points.
7. *Marking.* The marks made for the measurements should be discreet and of quality. For this, the use of black or white dermographic pencil is recommended, depending on the subject's skin tone. The pencils should be stored in cold places so that the tip does not melt due to the effect of heat, and for making finer marks. The thickness of the marks should not exceed one millimetre, and these should be clean to have a good precision in the measurement. Upon completion, the subject's skin should be cleaned, especially the marks to which they do not have access. It is very important to take into account sociocultural aspects, and in the case of Islamic people, the skinfolds should not be marked with a cross; in this case, a "T" mark will be used.
8. *Language.* The anthropometrist should use the language agreed upon by the ISAK for references such as for example *acromiale, radiale, ...* This consideration is important to avoid the mistakes made throughout history, which have led to the use of incorrect measurements in the application of formulas for anthropometric calculations. It is also important to know colloquial terms and how to handle them correctly so that the patient/athletes can understand us because the subject does not always understand anatomical language. In conclusion, it is important to adapt the language to the subjects who are going to be measured.
9. *Oral hygiene.* The anthropometrist is going to be very physically close to the subject, so this is an aspect to consider for their comfort. The first recommendation is to maintain proper oral hygiene, with the use of chewing gum being advisable. These recommendations should especially be followed by people who smoke, have halitosis and/or consume coffee, as well as those who consume certain foods that can result in bad breath. It is important not to consume foods that cause poor oral hygiene when measurements are going to be taken.
10. *Hand cleaning.* Hands should be washed before and after each measurement.
11. *Comments.* One must be very respectful and avoid making comments about the individual's physique, tattoos, scars, or clothing, and it is very necessary to protect their privacy.
12. *Companion.* It is highly recommended that the subject is accompanied by their father, mother, coach, teacher, or companion, especially if they are a minor. The anthropometrist may also opt to have an assistant, so in the event of an uncomfortable incident, there is always a witness to clarify the events

that occurred. In addition, there are certain behaviours that disappear in the presence of third parties.

13. *Positioning of the anthropometrist.* Some of the measurements will be taken near difficult or intimate areas and these should never be touched. For this, the anthropometrist will ask the subject to manipulate their own clothing to facilitate the measurements. In addition, there are measurements that require a certain invasion of the subject's personal space. If this approach is made from the front it can be very uncomfortable or intimidating for the subject, so the anthropometrist will position themselves laterally to the subject, except for some justified and protocolised exceptions, such as the measurement of stretch stature, waist circumference, etc.
14. *Clothing of the anthropometrist.* Caution should be taken with the type of clothing worn by the anthropometrist. Care should be taken to avoid uncomfortable or inappropriate situations, such as excessively open shirts or trousers that reveal the lower back when bending over. The best option is sports trousers or tight-fitting Lycra-based clothing. The clothing and the anthropometrist should not give off odours, so proper hygiene is recommended.
15. *Delivery of results.* It is important and necessary to provide the results at the end of the assessment. These results should be accompanied by an explanation and their interpretation.
16. *Confidentiality.* The anthropometrist must not disclose any personal data of the individuals being assessed without their express consent. This information must be protected, in accordance with the law (Data Protection Act), and only the person or people related to the measurement itself should have access to it, as indicated in the informed consent. The informed consent forms and the data should be archived in a secure place for the minimum period required by the body or institution that approved the protocol.
17. *Background of the subject to be measured.* Whenever an anthropometric assessment is to be carried out, the health status of the person to be assessed should be consulted, in order to be aware of possible problems that may arise during the assessment.

2.7 Recommendations on the Equipment and Place Where Measurements Are to Be Taken

1. *Cleaning of equipment.* The equipment should also be sanitised between measurements.
2. *Rooms.* Measurements should be taken in private, in a room, or a separate space, avoiding public places or transit areas.
3. *Temperature.* It should be comfortable for the subject. For this, self-perception can be used, because if the measurer is comfortable and at ease, the subject is probably cold, as they are not wearing clothes. Therefore, one way to subjectively control the temperature so that the subject is comfortable, is for the

measurer to be a little sweaty and feel a bit warm. In addition, you can ask, or perceive through external signs such as goosebumps or shivering.

4. *Safety during the assessment.* The material should be well calibrated and checked by the anthropometrist to avoid problems derived from malfunctions. Although this rarely occurs, there should be an action plan in case an emergency occurs during the assessment.

2.8 Considerations in Special Situations

Occasionally, when facing an anthropometric assessment, it is possible to encounter people who have injuries, a large amount of subcutaneous adipose tissue, extremely tense skin, or some kind of functional diversity, which can make it very difficult to take some measurements safely. In these cases, it is recommended to make a modification in the measurement technique that is easy to standardise and note it in the observations for future occasions. However, the principle that should guide decision-making in these cases, is to avoid taking any measurement that compromises the physical or emotional well-being of the subject.

Another of the problems that can arise in anthropometric assessments are difficulties in understanding due to language issues. This can be due to either a lack of knowledge of the language or difficulty in the communication process caused by functional diversity. In this situation, it is recommended to have the help of friends, family members or guardians of the person to be assessed, or even an interpreter. However, if the communication barrier cannot be overcome and the anthropometrist is not sure if the subject is capable of understanding the measurement protocol to which they are going to be subjected in sufficient depth, it is recommended not to carry it out to avoid uncomfortable situations.

As a key aspect, it must be remembered above all that absolute respect must be shown. Measurements are taken on people with emotions and feelings, and it is preferable not to take a skinfold if that is going to lead to the appearance of a conflict of modesty or ethics.

2.9 Questionnaire

1. The study of the spatial distances between people and their effect on interpersonal behaviour refers to:
   (a) Ethics.
   (b) Proxemics.
   (c) Haptics.
   (d) None of the above.
2. Personal distance is considered when it is:
   (a) Less than 45 cm.
   (b) More than 125 cm.

   (c) Between 46 and 120 cm.
   (d) Between 15 and 55 cm.
3. Ethical behaviour is characterised by:
   (a) Honesty, justice and fairness in interpersonal relationships.
   (b) Honesty, justice and fairness in professional relationships.
   (c) Honesty, justice and fairness in research and academic activities.
   (d) All are true.
4. Taking into account how sex, ethnicity and/or disability can have an influence is part of the ethical considerations regarding:
   (a) Who is going to be measured.
   (b) How it is going to be measured.
   (c) Where it is going to be measured.
   (d) When it is going to be measured.
5. The first step that should be taken when a subject is going to start an anthropometric evaluation is:
   (a) Sign the informed consent.
   (b) Explain the protocol that will be followed and the measurements that will be taken.
   (c) Ask them to stay alone with the necessary clothing for the measurement.
   (d) Provide information about the results of the measurements.
6. Regarding the clothing that subjects should wear, it is false that:
   (a) It should be indicated in advance of the measurement so that they can come prepared.
   (b) It should consist of shorts for men and a sports top and shorts for women.
   (c) In some cases, it is acceptable to take measurements in underwear.
   (d) Shorts can be replaced with a swimsuit and the sports top with a bikini.
7. Regarding the recommendations for anthropometrists, it is false that:
   (a) The use of appropriate language is not relevant.
   (b) Possible sociocultural differences should be taken into account.
   (c) The temperature of the room where the measurements are taken should be suitable for the subject being assessed.
   (d) Cleanliness, both of the equipment and the anthropometrist's hands, is an essential aspect.
8. When an anthropometric measurement is taken, the presence of a companion is advisable because:
   (a) It can help the subject being evaluated feel more comfortable.
   (b) Certain behaviours disappear in the presence of others.
   (c) If an uncomfortable event occurs, they can help clarify the facts.
   (d) All are true.
9. Regarding the confidentiality of the data:
   (a) It is advisable, but not essential, for there to be confidentiality of the subject's data.
   (b) The subject should not be informed about the treatment that will be carried out with their data.

(c) The subject's personal data are confidential and must be protected by law, so they cannot be published unless express authorisation from the subject is obtained.
(d) All are false.

10. Generally, during anthropometric measurements, it is true that:
    (a) It is recommended to avoid taking any action that compromises the physical or emotional well-being of the subject.
    (b) Respect must be shown, but it is more important to correctly carry out the protocol.
    (c) Data should be taken rigorously, even if the subject feels a little uncomfortable.
    (d) It is recommended to comply with the ethical considerations outlined, but they are not mandatory.

Answers:
1b, 2c, 3d, 4a, 5b, 6c, 7a, 8d, 9c, 10a.

Bibliography

Aragonés-Clemente, M. T., Casajús-Mallen, J. A., Rodríguez-Guisado, F., & Cabañas-Armesilla, M. D. (1993). Protocol of anthropometric measures. In E. Esparza (Ed.), *Manual of kinanthropometry* (pp. 35–66). FEMEDE.

Esparza-Ros, F., Vaquero-Cristóbal, R., & Marfell-Jones, M. (2019). *International protocol for anthropometric assessment*. International Society for the Advancement of Kinanthropometry.

Hollings, S. C., & Hume, P. A. (2018). Training and accreditation systems and ethical considerations. In P. Hume, D. A. Kerr, &, T. R. Ackland (Eds.), *Best practice protocols for physique assessment in sport* (pp. 231–241). Springer.

Anthropometric Equipment and Its Characteristics

3

Abstract

This chapter details the equipment necessary to carry out anthropometric measurements accurately and reliably. The equipment required to mark the subject before the measurements is listed, including an anthropometric box, a dermographic pencil, wet wipes, a segmometer and an anthropometric measuring tape. The instruments necessary for the measurement itself, such as the weighing scale, the stadiometer, the arm span equipment, the skinfold caliper, the anthropometric measuring tape, the small sliding caliper and the large sliding caliper are also described. The characteristics and recommendations for the use of each equipment are detailed, as well as the verification conditions to ensure the accuracy of the measurements. Alternatives and specific considerations for each tool are discussed, as well as the choice between manufacturing materials, verification methods and adjustment, and recommendations to maintain the durability and reliability of the equipment. Finally, the importance of maintaining accurate records of the measurements made, both in electronic and manual format, to provide detailed reports on the anthropometric characteristics of the subjects measured and to monitor evolution over time, is indicated

Keywords

Anthropometric equipment • Anthropometric box • Skinfold caliper • Segmometer • Anthropometric measuring tape • Small sliding caliper • Large sliding caliper • Weighing scale • Stadiometer • Arm span equipment

© The Author(s), under exclusive license to Springer Nature Switzerland AG 2025

F. Esparza-Ros and R. Vaquero-Cristóbal, *Anthropometry*,
https://doi.org/10.1007/978-3-031-77535-2_3

3.1 Necessary Equipment to Perform an Anthropometric Measurement

When performing an anthropometric measurement, the first thing that must be done is to mark the subject, and for this, the following anthropometric equipment is needed:

- Anthropometric box.
- Dermographic pencil or eyeliner.
- Wet wipes or makeup remover.
- Segmometer.
- Anthropometric measuring tape.

Once the subject is marked, the equipment necessary for the measurement are as follows:

- Weighing scale, for the measurement of body mass.
- Stadiometer, for the measurement of stretch stature and sitting height.
- Arm span equipment, for the measurement of the arm span.
- Skinfold caliper, for the measurement of skinfolds.
- Anthropometric measuring tape, for the measurement of girths.
- Small sliding caliper, for the measurement of small breadths.
- Large sliding caliper, for large breadths.

During the measurement and at the end of it, the following equipment will also be necessary:

- Record sheet

Furthermore, all anthropometric equipment must be regularly verified. The importance of verifying the equipment lies in the fact that it cannot be assumed that the equipment always measures accurately due to wear and tear from use.

Next, the equipment that needs to be used for the measurements is described.

3.1.1 Anthropometric Box

This is an important piece of equipment for making reliable measurements and achieving excellent ergonomics, both for the measurer and the person being measured. The dimensions of the box are: 40 cm high, 50 cm wide and 30 cm deep, which provides three different heights depending on the side that is placed against the floor, allowing the box to be used in different positions to perform the anthropometric measurements depending on the stature of the person to be measured. It is necessary that all sides be solid, since, depending on the stretch stature of the person, he/she will be placed at a height of 30 cm if it is for seating an infant and keeping their knees at 90°, at a height of 40 cm if it is for seating an adult, and at a height of 50 cm if it is for seating a very tall person. But the box can also be used to raise the subject or for the anthropometrist to step up in case the differences in heights or perspectives between both subjects do not allow some marking or measurement to be made ergonomically and reliably.

In addition, the box should have a cut-out section on at least one of its sides, this being necessary for the measurement of certain heights included in the full ISAK profile. Similarly, it is advisable for the box to have handles, because the box itself serves as a transport case in which we can introduce the anthropometric equipment.

The price of the box varies depending on the material chosen for its manufacturing (cardboard or wood). The main advantage of the wooden box over the cardboard one is durability, but its main disadvantage is weight. Therefore, if a wooden box is chosen, it is advisable that the wood not be excessively heavy, as this will make it difficult to transport. In this sense, boat wood is recommended. If a carpenter manufactures the box, it is recommended to check the measurements of the box when collecting it.

3.1.2 Dermographic Pencil or Eyeliner

It is essential that the dermographic pencil or eyeliner used allows for easy erasure of the marks made, as the subjects being measured should leave the consultation in the same conditions in which they arrived.

The dermographic pencil or eyeliner has the advantage of being easily erased, but the disadvantage of breaking easily when the temperature is high. Therefore, the pencils should be kept in a cool place and a sharpener should be used to keep the tip sharp. It is advisable to keep them in the fridge, in geographical areas where the ambient temperature is high.

An alternative to the dermographic pencil or eyeliner is the use of washable markers, which also easily erased with wet wipes, although their use is somewhat less professional than in the case of the pencil.

3.1.3 Wet Wipes or Makeup Remover

The importance of this equipment lies in the professionalism and quality it brings to the anthropometric measurement process, as it offers the subject the possibility of erasing the marks at the end of the measurement, with help provided for erasing the marks to which the subject does not have access.

3.1.4 Segmometer

Its use is limited in the restricted profile of the ISAK to the making of two anthropometric marks: the mid acromiale-radiale and thigh skinfold. Its limited utility, coupled with its high price, makes it a dispensable instrument for an ISAK level 1 anthropometrist. However, it is an interesting instrument for the two mentioned marks of the ISAK level 1, especially for the making of the thigh skinfold, as it requires access to very intimate areas, and with the segmometer it is not necessary to be so invasive. Thus, for the measurement of these marks, its utility lies in that it grants a greater quality to the measurement, as well as more proximity, with this being especially important in modest populations such as infants or some groups of adults. This instrument becomes indispensable when there is a need to measure lengths and heights with the necessary precision (full profile of the ISAK protocol).

Regarding the characteristics of the segmometer, it features a steel measuring tape that is 150 cm long and 15 mm wide, with two straight arms that are 7–8 cm in length. The division of the instrument is 1 mm. It should be noted that it should not be used to measure large bone breadths, as the tape deforms when pressure is applied.

For its verification, an anthropometric measuring tape or a Vernier caliper is used, although this instrument rarely loses adjustment.

3.1.5 Anthropometric Measuring Tape

The anthropometric measuring tape is used as auxiliary equipment for making some anthropometric marks, for measuring girths, as well as for verifying other anthropometric equipment. The main characteristic of this instrument is that it must be metallic, made of steel, preventing it from deforming when used and introducing error in the measurements. Therefore, the anthropometric measuring tape cannot be extendable, but it must be flexible to allow making adapt to the shape of the different areas in the measurement of girths. In addition, before starting the numbering, it must present at least three centimetres without numbering, so that when the tape is gripped to measure the girths, the reading of the girth is not covered with the fingers.

The minimum length of the tape is one and a half metres, although most have two metres to be able to verify the stadiometer and the arm span equipment. The measurements are obtained in centimetres, with graduation in millimetres, and with a division of its scale of 1 mm. It features an automatic retraction system that allows the tape to be collected automatically, facilitating the measurement to the anthropometrist. It is important to note the importance of storing the tape in its box to increase its durability.

For the verification of the anthropometric tape, the Vernier caliper is used. Although the anthropometric tape does not usually become damaged, the spring that allows the automatic retraction loses efficiency with use and may eventually break. In addition, over the years, the numbers lose sharpness, making reading difficult and therefore preventing it, or may even be erased, requiring the replacement of the tape.

3.1.6 Anthropometric Weighing Scale

The anthropometric weighing scale allows for the measurement of body mass and should have a division of its scale between 50 and 100 g. It is common for its scale to be 100 g, and it should allow a minimum measurement of 120 kg. Electronic weighing scales are recommended because they are easy to transport. Other types of weighing scales such as Roman weighing scales have the disadvantages of having limited transportability and requiring more time and training for taking a measurement.

The verification of the weighing scale is essential at least once a year. Specifically, for the verification of the anthropometric weighing scale, calibration weights are used to determine if the weighing scale continues to weigh correctly.

3.1.7 Stadiometer

The stadiometer allows us to measure the stretch stature and sitting height. It is advisable that it is fixed to the wall and on hard, stable, and level ground. However, the straightness of the wall should be checked, because if it presents any alteration it can induce an error in the measurement. A recommended feature that the stadiometer should include is a piece at the top that rests on the wall and allows it to remain straight when the subject being measured leans on the stadiometer to take the measurement.

Regarding the recommended characteristics of this instrument, it is necessary that it has a movable rod that is at least 6 cm wide with a locking device, which allows it to be placed on the vertex once the measurement manoeuvre has been carried out and, subsequently locked, remaining fixed at that height, allowing the subject being measured to leave the stadiometer and facilitate the reading of the height by the anthropometrist.

Stadiometers measure between 60 and 220 cm and have a division of their scale of 1 mm.

The verification of this instrument will depend on the type of stadiometer. Certain models require virtually no verification beyond checking that the pieces still fit well and that they have not lost their verticality, while other models require that at the time of installation, the anthropometrist ensures that the stadiometer is correctly adjusted and that the measurement truly starts from where the scale does. The verification of this instrument includes the measurement of the distance of the stadiometer with a tape measure, as well as the operation of the brake or gear.

Stadiometers that include a weighing scale are not recommended because they have a spring system at the base of the weighing scale that wears out over time, introducing error in the measurement, and also tends to lean backwards because it does not have the upper rod that allows it to remain straight.

An alternative to the use of a stadiometer is a ruler fixed to the wall, although it is necessary to verify that it is completely vertical. This can be checked using a level and the anthropometric measuring tape. As a complement to the tape fixed to the wall, it is necessary to have a 90° square to act as a rod in the measurement of stretch stature and sitting height.

3.1.8 Arm Span Equipment

This instrument is usually used for the measurement of specific populations in which arm span is a relevant indicator of performance.

There are alternatives to the common arm span equipment measurement that are more commonly used. The main alternative is the use of a square next to a metre fixed to the wall. It must have a minimum length of 220 cm to cover any type of population, and it is necessary to place one of the ends next to a corner. This method must be completed with a 90° square to measure how far the middle finger (dactylion) reaches on the tape measure that has fixed stuck to the wall, with the other dactylion touching to the corner wall.

For the validation of this instrument or its alternatives, a tape measure is used, ensuring that the tape measure fixed to the wall is straight with a level, in case this method is used.

3.1.9 Skinfold Caliper

The skinfold caliper is used for measuring skinfolds. This instrument can be made of metal, including a dial, or plastic. Among the characteristics of skinfold calipers, it is noteworthy that all must exert the same pressure (10 gr/mm^2), with this value being chosen based on a research study conducted in which it was observed that the pressure of the plates influenced the thickness of the measured skinfold and the consistency and the reproducibility of the measurement, finding a great reproducibility of repeated skinfolds when the pressure used was between 9 and 20 gr/mm^2. The spring presents hysteresis or the ability to retain its properties when the stimulus ceases to be exerted, so when the spring is stretched it presents some resistance at the time of returning to its initial position, causing the pressure exerted throughout the travel to not be exactly 10 gr/mm^2, but it is 10 ± 0.5 gr/mm^2. For this reason, the lower range (10 gr/mm^2) was sought so that the skinfolds were reproducible and it was not necessary to exert more pressure.

As an alternative to dial skinfold calipers, we find durable plastic skinfold calipers. This instrument has a division of its scale of 0.5 mm, which is smaller as compared to the division of the dial skinfold caliper which is between 0.1–0.2 mm, but it is a sufficiently reliable reading for anthropometric assessment with subjects who do not participate in high level sports. The main advantages of plastic skinfold calipers over dial ones are their price and durability, as the dial ones are more fragile due to the glass that covers the dial. In addition, plastic skinfold calipers have proven to be scientifically valid and reliable, showing a similar understanding and reading capacity as the dial ones, with a measurement range of 80 mm, being the most recommended for the majority of anthropometrists. Among the limitations present in the plastic skinfold calipers are the need for adaptation during the positioning and handling, and that they do not have a mechanism to exert the same pressure throughout the movement, which decreases the division as compared to the dial ones. This makes the margin of pressure in these skinfold calipers to be 10 ± 1 gr/mm^2, with this being within the permissible limits for the instrument to be valid and reliable. For all the above, plastic skinfold calipers are a great alternative for most anthropometrists, although the exception to the above may be when the skinfold calipers are used in research studies in which a large division of the scale is required, where it is advisable to have reference marks, or when working with elite athletes and there is a need for the skinfold caliper scale to be as precise as possible. Another alternative that has been greatly developed in recent years is the digital skinfold caliper. This type of skinfold caliper works with an application that performs the reading of the skinfold automatically, which is then recorded in the application, eliminating the reading and transmission error between the measurer and recorder. This type of skinfold caliper has shown to provide a reading similar to that of analogue skinfold calipers. They are, therefore, another useful alternative to consider when acquiring a skinfold caliper.

All metal and plastic skinfold calipers have the same parts and the same mechanism. Thus, there is a handle by which the instrument is held, a fixed upper arm, a movable lower arm, which is opened to perform the measurement, and a dial or scale where you can see the separation in mm between the application faces of the arms, a value that will correspond to the thickness of the measured skinfold when a measurement is performed. The measurement range of the skinfold caliper is usually up to 40 mm; however, this may be insufficient for the measurement of people who are overweight or obese, so that for this population, the use of skinfold calipers with a range of 80 mm is recommended.

The verification of the skinfold caliper depends on whether the instrument is metal or plastic. In both cases, the properties of the spring must be verified every 12 months, in reference to the pressure exerted by the skinfold caliper, as well as the opening of the skinfold caliper every 6 months, or the alignment of the plates every 6 months. In the case of dial skinfold calipers, we must add that the adjustments need to be greased when necessary, that there is a need to check the deterioration of the plates periodically, and ensure that the dial is at zero at the time of starting each measurement.

There are different methods of verifying the pressure depending on whether it is done in the ascending phase (arms of the skinfold caliper opening) or descending (arms of the skinfold caliper closing), or whether it is done statically or dynamically. Thus, while there are methods for static ascending verification, such as anchoring the fixed arm of the skinfold caliper to a vertical device and then hanging weights from the mobile arm and seeing how they affect the opening of the plates, or static descending verification methods, such as using a pressure gauge starting from an open position of the plates to a closed position, the most important pressure verification method is verification with foam blocks, as it is the most similar to the movement that the skinfold caliper will make on the skin when compressing the adipocytes during an anthropometric measurement (dynamic descending scale). The foam block is the material that best represents what happens in the skin and adipocytes when we place the skinfold caliper to measure, as we observe deformation in the sponge until it stabilises.

To carry out this verification, foam blocks or sponges of different densities are needed, generally between 15 and 55 mm thick, to mimic all possible ranges of skinfolds that we can measure in a subject. Each foam block is marked to place the plates of the skinfold caliper always in the same position. It should be noted that the mark made on the sponge should not be placed near the ends of it, as the density is different, with the ideal place to mark being the centre of the sponge, or at least two centimetres from all the margins of the foam block. For verification, the plates of the skinfold caliper are placed on the mark made on the sponge, after which ten series of one repetition per foam block from thinner to thicker are performed, leaving a minute between each series. A real measurement with the skinfold caliper should be replicated, applying it at a 90° and reading its value after two seconds. If the mode of the values obtained is similar to the one obtained the previous year or when the skinfold caliper was first acquired, the instrument measures adequately and we only need to store the used sponges in a place where they are not exposed to light and are not compressed, as this can modify their shape or density and will not allow repeating the verification later.

However, the gold standard for the verification of skinfold calipers is a device in which a load cell has been coupled to a separation controller. This device allows the performance of an absolute verification, that is, both static and dynamic and both on an ascending and descending scale. However, it is not easy to manufacture and if purchased, its price is quite expensive, so the method of foam blocks has become the most popularly used and disseminated among anthropometrists.

In addition to the pressure, it is important to verify the opening of the skinfold caliper. For this, a Vernier caliper can be used, but it is difficult to be precise with this method. Therefore, a recommendation is made to perform the verification three times with calibration block that are 10 to 40 mm thick. It should be noted that the faces of the skinfold caliper in the opening are not parallel, but they open obliquely forming a certain angle, so it is essential to place the spacer on the inner face of the skinfold caliper plate to standardise the verification conditions. For the verification, two possibilities are presented: (a) measure the length of the calibration block with the anthropometric tape, and using the corrected formula of the sine angle, calculate what value the dial should give; or (b) use the calibration block at the moment in which the skinfold caliper was acquired, write down the value, and repeat this protocol every six months to ensure that it continues to measure adequately.

In the event that the measurements taken to verify the pressure or the opening of the skinfold caliper do not provide a value similar to the last verification, or when the skinfold caliper was acquired, the operation of the skinfold caliper may have been altered. In the case of plastic skinfold calipers, the only thing that can be altered is the operation of the spring. To check this, it will be necessary to remove the spring from the skinfold caliper and apply Hooke's Law. To do this, the spring is placed in a vertical position and a certain amount of weight is hanged from it, recording the distance it stretches, and subsequently, double the weight that was previously added, recording the distance it stretches again. If the spring stretches twice as much the second time compared to the first, it will indicate that the operation is correct, so an error may have been made in the verification process, which is not usually the most common finding. On the other hand, if the spring does not stretch twice the length in the second measurement as compared to the first measurement, but stretches more, it will indicate that it has deformed, making it necessary to replace the spring with another of the same breadth and length.

However, in metal skinfold calipers with an analogue dial, it is not only the spring that may have broken, as it could be the mechanism within the skinfold caliper used to exert a constant pressure, or the dial. In case the spring is in perfect condition, but the skinfold caliper marks a different value than that of previous verifications, the dial must be moved to correct the error that the skinfold caliper is making when the measurement is taken with it.

3.1.10 Small Sliding Caliper

The small sliding caliper is used for the measurement of small bone breadths. The main difference between the small sliding caliper and the Vernier caliper is that the arms of the small sliding caliper are longer to allow it to be placed on the most medial and lateral part of the bones when they have a certain depth, as is the case with the condyles of the femur.

Regarding the characteristics of the small sliding caliper, it should present a scale of at least 15 cm, long arms of at least 10 cm, application face of 1.5 cm and resolution of 1 mm.

Similar to skinfolds calipers, the small sliding caliper can be made of metal or plastic. The main difference between them is the price, with the metal one being more expensive. However, the plastic small sliding caliper presents validity and reliability for making the measurement, only requiring a greater maintenance, as it requires oil from time to time so that the movement is fluid, and an adjustment of the pressure of the screws.

For its verification, a tape measure or a Vernier caliper is used.

3.1.11 Large Sliding Caliper

The large sliding caliper is used to measure the large breadths included in the full ISAK profile. The most interesting models are those that include straight arms to measure all breadths and antero-posterior abdominal depth, but also include curved arms or in the shape of an L or C to measure the antero-posterior chest depth.

When using a large sliding caliper with both types of arms, the appropriate scale must be read, since the reading will differ when the "L" shaped arms are introduced, from the one made when the straight arms are used, as the distance between the application faces of the "L" is less than between the straight arms. Because of this, this type of large sliding caliper usually includes two scales, one for measuring the distance from straight arm to straight arm of the large sliding caliper, while the other measures the distance between the application face of the "L" shaped arms. In other cases, the large sliding caliper does not have two scales, so it is necessary to manually subtract the length of both "L" branches from the measurement taken. In case of doubt, the reported measurement can always be checked by measuring the distance between arms with the anthropometric tape, and checking that the value matches the one reported on the scale.

The verification of the large sliding caliper is carried out with a tape measure, although it is not as determinant as with other instruments, for example with small sliding calipers, as they are much more durable materials, whose only nuance is the need to carry a screwdriver kit in case it is necessary to adjust some of their gears. In addition, it is true that they require a certain amount of maintenance, as with use, the movement becomes less fluid, although this instrument includes a screw mechanism with which the fluidity of the slide can be adjusted. In addition, it may be necessary to use oil every so often to facilitate movement.

3.1.12 Record Sheet

During the measurement process and at the end of it, with the aim of being able to analyse the results of the anthropometric measurement and provide the measured subject with a report on their anthropometric characteristics and derived variables (body composition, somatotype and proportionality) a record sheet and anthropometric *software* that is filled out simultaneously on a computer and by hand.

The electronic record sheet or anthropometric software allows the anthropometrist to provide the subject with a report as soon as the measurement is finished, which indicates how they have changed as compared to the previous measurement, or in case it is the first measurement, indicate the goal to achieve based on their starting point, or in comparison to a reference group or subject.

However, the electronic record has a drawback, which is the risk of the device we are making the notes on turning off or the file being deleted. For this reason, filling out a manual record is recommended in parallel to the electronic record, to avoid the loss of the data entered on the electronic sheet. However, the availability of an assistant to carry out the parallel recording will be necessary. In case of not having an assistant to carry out the manual record, the computer program can be configured to perform an automatic save every minute.

3.2 Tips for Using Anthropometric Equipment

Finally, there are a series of tips regarding the use of anthropometric equipment that should be taken into consideration:

- Check the condition of the equipment before proceeding with the measurement.
- Use different magnitudes for verification.
- Look for and use reference instruments that meet the specified characteristics.
- For the research field, the quality, accuracy and division of the equipment is important.
- Replace deteriorating parts periodically, and follow the manufacturer's advice for storing the material.
- Check the proper functioning of the equipment before and after its use.

3.3 Questionnaire

1. Indicate which of the following equipment is NOT necessary for marking the subject before measurement:
   (a) Segmometer.
   (b) Anthropometric tape.
   (c) Stadiometer.
   (d) Anthropometric box.
2. Which of the following instruments is used for the assessment of bone breadths?
   (a) Small sliding caliper.
   (b) Skinfold caliper.
   (c) Segmometer.
   (d) Anthropometric tape.
3. Regarding the verification of the equipment used in anthropometric measurements, indicate the true statement:
   (a) The equipment should be verified only the first time it is used.
   (b) The equipment is factory calibrated and does not need to be checked for verification at any time.
   (c) The use and wear of the equipment can cause it to become uncalibrated, so it should be checked regularly.
   (d) None of the above is true.
4. Indicate the false statement regarding the anthropometric box:
   (a) It is a very important piece of equipment to maintain the ergonomics of the measurer and the subject.

   (b) The dimensions are not important as long as it is sturdy and stable.
   (c) It should have a section cut out on one of its sides, necessary for the measurement of some heights in the complete ISAK profile.
   (d) It can serve as a transport box for the anthropometric equipment.
5. The anthropometric tape (indicate the false statement):
   (a) It is used in the measurement of muscle girths.
   (b) It should be metallic and flexible, but not extendable.
   (c) The total minimum length should be at least 1.5 m.
   (d) It is a dispensable material that can be replaced by others.
6. Among the characteristics of the anthropometric weighing scale, we find:
   (a) The division of its weighing scale should be between 50 and 100 g.
   (b) It is advisable that it allows measurements up to 120 kg or more.
   (c) Electronic weighing scales are recommended for their ease of transport and the wide range of prices that can be found.
   (d) All of the above are true.
7. Regarding skinfold calipers, indicate the false answer:
   (a) They are used for the measurement of skinfolds.
   (b) The pressure they exert is not considered relevant and does not affect the measurement of the skinfolds.
   (c) Depending on the model, they usually have a division of their scale between 0.5 and 0.1 mm.
   (d) Plastic skinfold calipers with a spring system are a valid and reliable alternative to dial ones, despite having a smaller scale division.
8. Regarding the verification of the skinfold calipers:
   (a) The pressure exerted by the spring should be checked at least every 12 months.
   (b) Only the pressure should be checked, as the opening and alignment of the plates does not vary.
   (c) There is no standardised method for measuring the pressure exerted by a skinfold caliper.
   (d) All of the above are true.
9. Indicate the correct answer regarding the small sliding caliper:
   (a) It is used to measure girths.
   (b) It is similar to a Vernier caliper, but with longer arms to facilitate its use.
   (c) Currently, only metal-made small sliding calipers are valid.
   (d) Due to its characteristics, it does not need verification.
10. Regarding the record sheets:
   (a) It is exclusively recommended to keep the record in electronic format as it has no drawbacks.
   (b) If the anthropometrist has a good memory, the record sheet can be filled out once the measurement has been completed.
   (c) The electronic record sheet or anthropometric software allows us to analyse the data and provide the report to the subject as soon as the measurement is finished.
   (d) None of the above is true.

Answers:
1.c 2.a 3.c 4.b 5.d 6.d 7.b 8.a 9.b 10.c

Bibliography

Esparza-Ros, F., Vaquero-Cristóbal, R., & Marfell-Jones, M. (2019). *International protocol for anthropometric assessment*. International Society for the Advancement of Kinanthropometry.

Geeta, A., Jamaiyah, H., Safiza, M. N., Khor, G. L., Kee, C. C., Ahmad, A. Z., Suzana, S., Rahmah, R., & Faudzi, A. (2009). Reliability, technical error of measurements and validity of instruments for nutritional status assessment of adults in Malaysia. *Singapore Medical Journal, 50*(10), 1013–1018.

Lohman, T. G., & Pollock, M. L. (1981). Skinfold measurement: Which caliper? How much training? *Journal of Physical Education and Recreation, 52*, 27–29.

Orphanidou, C., McCargar, L., Birmingham, C. L., Mathieson, J., & Goldner, E. (1994). Accuracy of subcutaneous fat measurement: Comparison of skinfold calipers, ultrasound, and computed tomography. *Journal of the American Dietetic Association, 94*(8), 855–858.

Sources of Error and Statistics Applied to Anthropometry

4

Abstract

This chapter addresses the importance of accuracy and precision in anthropometric measurements, highlighting how measurement errors can affect the interpretation of results. Various sources of error are mentioned, including challenges related to the measurement technique, environmental conditions, the biological variability of individuals, the verification of the equipment used, and the reading and recording of data. The need to follow standardised protocols to minimise error is emphasised, as well as the importance of training and familiarisation with the equipment used. In addition, specific recommendations are provided to reduce measurement errors, such as taking multiple measurements of the same variable and maintaining a suitable environment for measurements. The second part of the chapter specifies how to perform the error analysis in anthropometry. Thus, it delves into the concepts of precision (intra-evaluator technical measurement error), validity, accuracy (inter-evaluator technical measurement error) and probability of success (confidence intervals), as well as the calculations for each of them and the interpretation of the results.

Keywords

Precision • Accuracy • Sources of error • Technical measurement error • Probability of success • Standardisation

4.1 Introduction

The importance of knowing whether a measurement is precise and accurate begins with the quantification of the possible error made during the measurement, on which the truthfulness of the results will depend when communicating the changes produced in the subject analysed, or the differences found between it and a reference population. Thus, it is possible that the differences between measurements or

© The Author(s), under exclusive license to Springer Nature Switzerland AG 2025
F. Esparza-Ros and R. Vaquero-Cristóbal, *Anthropometry*,
https://doi.org/10.1007/978-3-031-77535-2_4

populations are real, or that they are due to the evaluator's margin of error when taking the measurement.

In this regard, it is important to bear in mind that the anthropometric method may seem deceptively simple, but this method is only useful when a series of guidelines and protocols are taken into account, to maintain its validity through the quality of the measurement, the achievement of which is one of the foundations of anthropometry. Thus, it is essential that the margin of error in the anthropometrist's measurement is minimal in order to provide the highest quality to the measurement taken. To achieve this goal, it is important to control possible sources of error.

The error may come because the measurement techniques and conditions are not being followed, because the individual we are measuring has undergone some type of biological variation, because the material is not correctly verified, or because some type of error is being made in the reading and recording of the data.

4.2 Possible Sources of Error Regarding the Technique and Measurement Conditions

In order to reduce the error derived from a poor establishment of the technique and measurement conditions, it must be taken into account that the measurement technique is standardised and this protocol must be followed, that it is necessary to make several measurements of the same variable to reduce the random error of the measurer (anthropometrist) when taking the variable, that work must be done with a recorder (troika) and that the measurement must be made under certain space conditions.

4.2.1 Standardised Technique

One of the most frequent sources of error in anthropometric measurements is the lack of standardisation in the measurements taken or failures when applying the protocol. In this regard, the International Society for the Advancement of Kinanthropometry (ISAK) has established a very meticulous standardised protocol for both the making of anthropometric marks and the taking of measurements, with adherence to these guidelines being fundamental to minimize error in the anthropometric assessment of an individual. In this way, it ensures that measurements are always taken under the same conditions, using the same technique, and therefore allows for the comparison of test results, whether in tracking progress or in cross-sectional data comparison.

Below are some of the most common errors:

- Taking the abdominal skinfold horizontally, when it should be taken vertically.
- Taking the thigh skinfold with the subject's knee bent, when this skinfold is taken with the knee fully extended and the heel on the ground.

- Taking the subscapular skinfold in the wrong direction. In this regard, the subscapular skinfold is taken at a 45° oblique angle downwards and outwards from the subscapulare point, which is at the lower angle of the lower part of the scapula. This is done following the direction marked according to the arrangement of the adipocytes and the natural lines of the skin.
- Taking measurements without having previously marked (painted). If this is done, it cannot be ensured that future measurements will be taken in the same place, and whether that place is appropriate.
- Taking two or three measurements of the same variable consecutively. Doing this may influence the second and third measurements taken by the anthropometrist, based on the value found in the first measurement. Moreover, it does not give the tissues, especially the adipose tissue, time to return to their basal state before taking the second and/or third measurement.
- Taking the skinfold with the fingers "in pliers", or "duck beak", instead of "in clamp" or "parrot beak".
- Taking the skinfold with the fingers holding it at an angle to the body and not perpendicular to the mark made.
- Taking the skinfold with the fingers or the skinfold caliper on top of the cross when the fingers should be adjacent just before the cross and the skinfold caliper should enter one centimetre underneath.

If the standardised protocols presented are not followed, an error is introduced into the measurement and its validity is reduced.

4.2.2 Spaces for Taking Measurements

An anthropometric assessment should always be carried out in a private, noise-free room, where the anthropometrists can concentrate, where they can measure the person, and where the person has the privacy needed to carry out an anthropometric assessment. Under no circumstances should a measurement be taken in a noisy context or in a space where the subject we are measuring is exposed to uncomfortable situations due to the presence of colleagues or others. However, it is not recommended to take measurements alone, as it is always advisable to have an assistant present during the measurement to act as a note-taker, which can be requested from a member of the technical staff, a teacher, etc. In the case of minors, the presence of a parent/guardian is advised, as this provides a guarantee of transparency for all parties involved. In the informed consent, it is advisable to include a request for the parents/guardians of minors to accompany the measurements. In this way, the minor will be more relaxed, and the process will denote transparency to the relatives.

The subject should avoid exercising on the day the measurement is to be taken, before it, as there is swelling in the tissue and dehydration after sports practice, causing physiological changes that affect anthropometric variables, especially the measurement of girths. Also, in case of sweating, the skin does not present the appropriate conditions for carrying out the measurement. As a strategy, in the case of younger subjects, provide a board game or some form of entertainment to avoid activity prior to the measurement, in case they are waiting in an adjoining room; although the best solution is to gradually schedule the subjects based on the estimated measurement time to avoid waiting for either party.

4.2.3 Working in a Troika

It is recommended to work in a troika when carrying out anthropometric measurements. This means that the people involved in the measurement are: the anthropometrist, the subject to be measured, and the recorder/assistant. The latter is in charge of recording each of the measurements, but can also assist the anthropometrist in some of the measurements, especially in the case of large girths to ensure correct placement of the tape parallel to the ground during the measurement. If an assistant is not available, the placement of a mirror can provide a viewpoint from the side opposite the anthropometrist.

4.2.4 Performing Multiple Measurements

Anthropometry is a science in which the anthropometrist has a large percentage of influence over the final result reported. Therefore, and in order to reduce random error, it is necessary to perform multiple measurements of the same variable. If only one measurement is taken, it is very likely to be incorrect. It has been shown that by performing two measurements and taking their average as the final value, the measurement error can be reduced by up to 29.3%. In the meantime, if three measurements are taken and the median is used as the final value, the error can be reduced by up to 42.3%. For this reason, it is necessary to perform two or three measurements depending on whether the difference between them is greater than 5% in the skinfolds or 1% in the rest of the measurements.

The proper way to take these multiple measurements would be, once all the anatomical marks have been made on the subject, to perform a first measurement of all variables following the order established by the ISAK; after which a second measurement should be taken following the same order of all the variables. Finally, third measurements are taken for those variables where necessary.

There is a bad practice to avoid, which consists of taking the same measurement two or even three times in a row. Instinctively, it is usually assumed that the first measurement is correct, when it may not be. Therefore, the protocol indicates performing all the measurements in order, and once the first measurements are finished, repeat the process for the second and/or third. An important factor to consider regarding this bad practice is that when taking skinfolds, the pressure exerted produces a deformation on the adipose tissue. In the case of taking the same skinfold measurement twice in a row, the adipose tissue measured in the second measurement will not be in the same conditions as in the first case, whereas leaving a brief time between measurements, that adipose tissue recovers its initial state.

Therefore, the protocol to follow with a subject is:

- Signing of informed consent.
- Making marks on the subject.
- Taking the first measurement.
- Taking the second measurement.
- Taking the third measurement (when necessary).

On this last point, it would be ideal to perform a third measurement of all variables in order to greatly reduce the random error, but this would make the anthropometric assessment too long. This is the reason why the ISAK established that after performing the 2nd measurement of the same variable in a non-consecutive manner, if the difference between both measurements is greater than 5% for the skinfolds or 1% for the rest of the measurements, a third measurement should be taken, and the median of the three measurements should be used as the final value. The use of the median allows the elimination of extreme values without affecting the final result. On the contrary, if such a difference between the first two measurements is not found, it is assumed that the random error is minimal and a third measurement is not needed, using the average of both measurements made as the final value.

Therefore, the first thing to do is to know the difference between the first two measurements taken of a variable in order to, depending on the percentage of error between them, know if it is necessary to take a third measurement of that variable. The formula applied to find the percentage difference between the first two measurements is: (value 1st measurement − value 2nd measurement)/average of the 1st and 2nd measurements. For example: The subscapular skinfold of a subject was measured on two occasions. The first was 15.2 mm and the second 16 mm. The difference between both measurements is 0.8 mm. The average of both measurements is $(15.2 + 16)/2 = 15.6$. Therefore, $(0.8/15.6) * 100 = 5.13\%$ error between both measurements. As it is a skinfold, the margin of error that indicates the need for a third measurement is 5%. As the figure obtained is higher, a third measurement will have to be taken and the final value will be the median of the three measurements.

In the case of not having software that automates this process and the data are taken without this help, some guidelines will need to be followed to find if a third measurement is necessary. Regarding basic measurements, it is not usual to require a third measurement as only a 1% difference is allowed. Thus, regarding the body mass of a person that weighs 50 kg (average of 1st and 2nd measurements), the difference would have to be 0.5 kg or more between measurements. As for stretch stature and arm span, for a person who is 180 cm in stretch stature (average of 1st and 2nd measurements), the difference would have to be 1.8 cm or more between the measurements, which is not usual. For sitting height, for a person who measures 90 cm (average of 1st and 2nd measurements), the difference between measurements would have to be 0.9 cm or more for a third measurement (Table 4.1).

On the other hand, making third measurements is much more common in the other blocks of measurements. When we measure the skinfolds, with a skinfold caliper that has a precision of 0.5 mm, and the measurement is less than 10 mm, any variation between the first and second measurement will require a third measurement when the difference exceeds 5%. If the skinfold is between 10 and 20 mm, and the difference between the first and the second is 0.5 mm, a third measurement will not have to be taken. In the skinfolds greater than 20 mm, a 1 mm difference between the measurements taken is allowed. Thus, if the measurements are, for example, 23 mm in the first measurement, and 24 mm in the second measurement, a third measurement would not have to be taken (Table 4.1).

In the rest of the measurements (girths, lengths and heights, breadths and depths) the allowed margin is the value in millimetres as the measured variable in centimetres. For example, the margin of error of a variable such as the arm

Table 4.1 When to make a third measurement of a variable (manual calculations)

Variable	Value (mm)	Difference between first and second measurement in order to avoid taking a third measurement (mm)
Skinfolds	< 10	0
	≥ 10 to < 20	≤ 0.5
	≥ 20 to < 30	≤ 1
	≥ 30 to < 40	≤ 1.5
	≥ 40 to < 50	≤ 2
Other variables	0–9	0
	10–19	1
	20–29	2
	30–39	3
	40–49	4
	50–59	5
	60–69	6
	70–79	7
	80–89	8
	90–99	9
	100–109	10
	110–119	11
	120–129	12
	130–139	13
	140–149	14
	150–159	15

relaxed girth, where the average between the first two measurements is 30.4 cm (304 mm), is 3.0 mm. In a variable such as the hips girth, whose mean value is 101.9 cm (1019 mm), the margin of error would be 10.1 mm or 1.01 cm. In small breadths (humerus, bi-styloid, femur and bimalleolar), as these measurements are under 1 cm (it is not common to find values higher than 10 mm), there is no margin of error between the first and the second measurement, as the margin of error would be less than 1 mm, and the measurement scales are not precise enough (Table 4.1).

4.3 Possible Sources of Error Regarding the Individual's Biological Variation

The variability of the subjects can induce an error in the taking of anthropometric measurements. In this regard, it is necessary to take into account the time of day and the day of the week of the measurement, the stage of the menstrual cycle in the case of women of childbearing age, the performance of exercise prior to the measurement, the intake of large meals, the subject's body care (lotions, creams, etc. on the skin), the use of saunas, or biological variability. All of these factors can affect the level of hydration, skin turgor, tissue oedema or water retention, and can therefore influence the taking of anthropometric measurements.

4.3.1 Time of Day

There are certain anthropometric parameters that change throughout the day. Among them we find the decrease in stretch stature, due to the gradual loss of hydration of the intervertebral discs as a result of being upright, which can amount to 1 cm, so it will be necessary to note the time of measurement. The variation is also noticeable in the lower limb girths, resulting in oedema and vascularisation of the legs in subjects who spend long periods standing, increasing the leg girth throughout the day, especially in women as a result of usually having poorer venous return.

4.3.2 Day of the Week

When carrying out a longitudinal anthropometric follow-up on a person, it is advisable to take the measurements on the same day of the week, especially if it is an athlete. In any case, the day of the week when the evaluation is being carried out will have to be noted. This is due to the fact that people's weekly routine tends to be quite similar, but on the other hand, the daily routine tends to vary slightly, especially between weekdays and holidays, so this control minimises the error that may be produced. More specifically in the case of athletes, it is advisable to carry out the anthropometric assessment always after a rest day in which the athlete has not trained or competed, so that the results are not affected by the performance of physical exercise and the resulting oedema. In addition, carrying out the anthropometric assay the day after the rest day usually has a preventive effect on the performance of behaviours contrary to sports performance, such as heavy meals, intake of large amounts of alcohol or fast food, due to the belief that their behaviour on the day prior to the anthropometric measurement will affect the results, so that more suitable results to those expected will be obtained.

4.3.3 Menstrual Cycle

The stage of the menstrual cycle, in the case of fertile women, greatly affects hydration and skin elasticity, among other factors. While this can influence anthropometric variables, its effect might may not lie on the final result of the measurement, but on the difficulty in taking some variables such as skinfolds. On the contrary, the effect of the stage of the menstrual cycle on body composition assessed by anthropometry is less than that found when other techniques such as electrical bioimpedance are used, which are greatly influenced by the degree of hydration of the subject assessed.

4.3.4 Exercise

The practice of exercise produces an increase in oedema in the area involved, and as a result of this, the girth can increase. Therefore, an anthropometric assessment should not be carried out if the subject has previously exercised on the same day of the evaluation, unless the objective is precisely to assess the change produced in the girth by this phenomenon. Regardless of this factor, it is likely that the state of hydration after exercise is not the same as under basal conditions, so it will influence the taking of measurements. In addition, vigorous or high-intensity exercise should not be performed the day before, as part of the oedema of the area involved may continue when the measurement is taken. It is therefore ideal in the case of athletes to take the measurements after the rest day.

4.3.5 Heavy Meals

The intake of heavy meals should be avoided 24 h prior to the measurement, and especially in the mealtime prior to the measurement, due to its influence on the results of the anthropometric assessment. Specifically, this factor could contaminate the measurement of body mass and of girths such as the waist girth, among others.

4.3.6 Body Care

Special importance should be given to remind the subjects who are going to be measured not to wear oils or body creams. These will make the measurement difficult by causing the skinfold caliper to slip and the anthropometric tape to stick, introducing an error in the measurement. Although less common, this can also happen in people with oilier skin. Therefore, a pack of sanitary wipes and blotting paper should always be carried, so that in a situation where the skin is not in the right conditions, it can be cleaned and dried before taking the measurements.

4.3.7 Sauna

Exposure to saunas or environments with similar conditions can also cause changes in the level of hydration, affecting the elasticity of the skin and the girths. Therefore, exposure to this type of situations should be avoided 24 h prior to the measurement, to avoid factors that alter measurements such as skinfolds or girths.

4.3.8 Biological Variability

In a study conducted with cadavers in which they were anthropometrically assessed before being dissected (Martin et al., 1985), it was found that the pattern of adipose tissue showed a great intra and inter-subject variability in different body areas, with different compressibility, skin thickness and density of adipose tissue and skin. The skinfolds of the lower limb (thigh skinfold and leg skinfold) showed a lower compressibility, a low skin thickness, and a high correlation between the measurement of the skinfold and the amount of subcutaneous fat in the area when the dissection was performed. In spite of this, most of the formulas used for the estimation of adiposity do not include skinfolds of the lower limb. Two other conclusions from this article were that there are differences in the distribution of adiposity depending on sex, and that subcutaneous fat is not directly related to intramuscular adiposity. Due to these results, it is highly recommended to introduce in our studies the sum of six or eight skinfolds, and when an estimation of body composition is made, to choose a formula that includes skinfolds of the upper limbs, trunk, and lower limbs.

4.4 Possible Sources of Error Regarding Equipment Verification

Poor verification of equipment can be another source of error that decreases the reliability of the anthropometric measurement. In this sense, it is worth remembering that the anthropometrist must ensure the correct verification of the anthropometric material following the recommendations set out in the specific chapter.

4.5 Possible Sources of Error Regarding Data Reading and Recording

Errors can occur in the reading carried out by the anthropometrist, in the transmission of information from the anthropometrist to the recorder, or in the recorder's notation, with these errors influencing the anthropometric assessment. Below, some of the most common errors in this block are presented.

4.5.1 Reading Error

The reading error in the different measuring instruments used in anthropometry is another of the factors that can introduce an error in the measurement taken. Of the instruments used, skinfold calipers and large sliding calipers will introduce error more frequently.

As for the skinfold calipers, the ones that most frequently induce error are those that have an analogue dial for reading. The first error that should be avoided is that the dial should be at zero before making the measurement, so it is always necessary to check its position, which can sometimes be altered by unintentional manipulation by people unfamiliar with the technique. As for the type of dial and reading method, we must differentiate between the most popular brands, Harpenden and Holtain. On the face of the Harpenden dial the hands move in the direction of a clock hands, and it has a larger needle that indicates the measurement from 0 to 20 mm. Harpenden is capable of measuring up to 80 mm, and for this, it has a smaller dial, where a smaller hand indicates how many turns the main hand has made. Each turn of this small dial, tells us that we have to add 20 mm to those indicated by the larger hand. As for Holtain, the clock hand moves in the opposite direction to a clock hands. It has a dial skinfold caliper where the scale goes up to 40 mm. These characteristics of both skinfold calipers are frequent factors of reading error, so that remembering them frequently is necessary. On the other hand, digital skinfold calipers have the advantage of not requiring reading, which eliminates this source of error.

As for large sliding caliper, we must be careful when reading the antero-posterior chest depth to choose the correct scale, as the reading should be done on a different scale to the rest of the measurements.

In general, reading errors can be avoided with training and familiarisation with the equipment that is used regularly for anthropometric measurements.

4.5.2 Auditory Error

One of the most common errors in data recording is the auditory error that occurs at the time of transmission of the reading from the anthropometrist to the recorder and his/her reception of it. To avoid this error, the anthropometrist specifies the variable to be measured and then reads the result found unit by unit, indicating the decimal with "point". However, when entering it in the computer software, its configuration must be taken into account when writing the decimal of the measurement with a "." or with a ",". After this, the recorder will repeat aloud the value of the measurement he/she has heard before entering it, to confirm the correct reception of the information received. In this way the anthropometrist ensures that the recorder has received the indicated data correctly, facilitating communication between the anthropometrist and the recorder with each measurement. After this, the recorder indicates the next variable to be measured to the anthropometrist so that he/she does not have to think about what measurement comes next and waste the least possible time. This way of proceeding is very important in the third measurement, as the order of the measurement protocol is not usually followed, as a third measurement for all them is often not needed. In parallel, the recorder records the measurement on the written sheet and/or anthropometric software.

Below is an example of the above:

- Recorder says to the anthropometrist: "Arm relaxed girth".
- Anthropometrist says to the recorder: "Arm relaxed girth: three five point eight" (Reading: 35.8).
- Recorder: (repeats aloud) "Three five point eight" and then says the next measurement: "arm flexed and tensed girth" + notation of the arm relaxed girth on the sheet and/or software.

4.5.3 Measurement Placement Error

If the assistant is unfamiliar with the anthropometric technique, a placement error may occur in the annotations. This is because the assistant may not differentiate between skinfolds and girths when the anthropometrist indicates the measured area. For example, the anthropometrist might say "leg: three five point seven", and the recorder does not enter it in the leg, which is the body part measured, but the leg skinfold. To solve this, it is necessary to familiarise the recorder with the measurement sheet and give the annotator the complete information, specifying the block of variables that are going to be measured (basic measurements, skinfolds, girths, lengths and heights, or breadths and depths), and even if the variable is higher or lower on the list. In addition, the anthropometrist should review the recorded data once the evaluation has been completed to look for strange values in which this placement error may have occurred.

4.5.4 Transcription

It is also possible to find that there is a confusing transcription of the measurement annotated on paper. To try to avoid this source of error, in anthropometry, the annotation numbers have been standardised. In this way, zero is crossed out ("Ø"), one is a stick ("1"), four is made completely square ("4"), six is completely closed ("6"), seven has the horizontal stick ("7") and nine is completely closed ("9"). It is necessary for the recorder to make the annotation on paper and on the computer software simultaneously to try to identify any possible error in the annotation. This is because the error will persist if the measurements are entered in one of the two devices and then transcribed from one to another. Regarding the annotation in the computer software, the annotated data must be visually checked to avoid annotation errors on the keyboard.

4.6 Analysis of Errors in Anthropometry

Once the most common sources of error when performing an anthropometric assessment have been analysed, the concepts of precision, validity, accuracy and probability of success regarding the anthropometric assessment will be addressed next.

4.6.1 Precision—Intra-evaluator TEM

Precision is the variation observed in repeated measures carried out by the same anthropometrist on the same subject. It deals with the possibility that the measurements taken in similar circumstances and by the same anthropometrist resemble each other. The more similar the measurements in the same subject, in the same circumstances, the smaller the error of the anthropometrist. In addition, it should be noted that the precision of the anthropometrist is variable, specific, and is influenced by the characteristics and familiarisation of the anthropometrist with the population to be assessed.

Precision is calculated with the formula of the intra-evaluator technical error of measurement (TEM), which allows finding the variability that an evaluator shows when measuring a certain anthropometric variable repeatedly in a certain population. It is important for the biological variation of the individual not to influence the result obtained, that the two measurements that are going to be compared of each individual are taken in the same evaluation session, following the previously specified measurement protocol. For its calculation, it is necessary to include at least 20 subjects belonging to this population in order for the TEM found to be significant for it. The less variability shown in the final result of the intra-evaluator TEM in a given variable, the greater the precision of the evaluator in assessing that variable.

An important application of the calculation of the intra-evaluator TEM would be to be able to affirm whether the change that can be found in a measurement, as compared to previous ones taken from an individual, is due to an error by the anthropometrist in taking the measurement or due to the fact that the measurement had actually changed. Thus, for example, if, when calculating the intra-evaluator TEM, it is found that the error in the 8 skinfold sum of an anthropometrist in a certain population is 5 mm, and a subject changes his/her 8 skinfold sum by 3 mm between measurements, it cannot be affirmed that a change has occurred, since this change is within the margin of error that the anthropometrist makes in this variable and with specific population. If, on the other hand, the change shown by the subject was 10 mm, it could be affirmed with certainty that the skinfold value was reduced as the change is greater than the margin of error when the anthropometrist makes the measurement.

For the mathematical calculation of the intra-evaluator TEM, the following formula must be applied:

$$TEM = \sqrt{\frac{\Sigma d^2}{2n}}$$

Analysing it, the calculation of the intra-evaluator TEM will be carried out through the square root of the sum ($\sum$) of the squared differences of two measurements taken in the same variable from the same individual in the same evaluation session (d^2), divided by the product of two and the number of subjects from whom that variable was measured (n), including a pair of measurements from each subject. For example, if 20 subjects are measured, i.e. the first and second measurement of a certain variable, firstly the difference between the first and second measurement for each of the subjects is calculated; secondly, the difference found for each of the subjects is squared; thirdly, all the squared differences of the 20 subjects are added up; fourthly, the result is divided by 2 times the number of subjects, which in this case are 20; and fifthly and lastly, the square root of the resulting value from the previous division is made to find the intra-evaluator TEM.

Classically, for the calculation of the intra-evaluator TEM, the first two measurements were included, in the case that only two measurements had been made; and the two closest measurements, in the case that three measurements had been made.

Next, a numerical example of how to apply this is presented. An anthropometrist has measured 10 elite senior women handball players who present the following triceps skinfolds (mm) (Table 4.2).

The steps to be taken for the calculation of the intra-evaluator TEM are:

1. Difference between the first and second measurement for each of the subjects (Table 4.3).
2. The difference found for each of the subjects is squared (Table 4.4).
3. All the squared differences of the 10 subjects are added up (Table 4.5).
4. The result is divided by 2 times the number of subjects: $2.12/2 * 10 = 0.106$.

Table 4.2 Intra-evaluator TEM calculation: first and second measurements taken by the same anthropometrist

Subject	1	2	3	4	5	6	7	8	9	10
Measurement 1	9.9	8.6	11.6	10.3	11.7	9.9	10.8	9.4	7.6	8.8
Measurement 2	9.3	8.7	10.6	10.5	11.4	9.6	11.0	9.1	7.4	8.2

Table 4.3 Intra-evaluator TEM calculation: calculation of differences between first and second measurements taken by the same anthropometrist

Subject	1	2	3	4	5	6	7	8	9	10
Diff between measurement 1 and measurement 2	0.6	− 0.1	1.0	− 0.2	0.3	0.3	− 0.2	0.3	0.2	0.6

Table 4.4 Intra-evaluator TEM calculation: calculation of the square of the differences between the first and second measurements taken by the same anthropometrist

Subject	1	2	3	4	5	6	7	8	9	10
Diff^2	0.36	0.01	1.00	0.04	0.09	0.09	0.04	0.09	0.04	0.36

Table 4.5 Intra-evaluator TEM calculation: sum of squared differences between the first and second measurements taken by the same anthropometrist

Total subjects	10
Sum Diff^2	$0.36 + 0.01 + 1.00 + 0.04 + 0.09 + 0.09 + 0.04 + 0.09 + 0.04 + 0.36 = 2.12$

5. The square root of the resulting value is taken: $\sqrt{0.106} = 0.33\,\text{mm}$.

It should be noted that the intra-evaluator TEM decreases with experience in measuring. Therefore, its calculation is recommended every six months in the case of novice anthropometrists, as it is likely that their intra-evaluator TEM will significantly decrease in the first months and years of measurement, which will reduce the necessary margin of change in the measured subject to be able to affirm with certainty that it has changed significantly.

However, the absolute calculated intra-evaluator TEM does not allow the anthropometrist to conclusively know in which variables he/she is having a greater margin of error, as the absolute intra-evaluator TEM cannot be compared between different variables as they do not present similar values. Seen another way, for the same intra-evaluator TEM, the smaller the value of the measured value, the greater percentage of error it will represent within the variable, and therefore, the more it will be influencing its final result. In order to know the percentage of error of the anthropometrist when measuring a certain variable in a specific population, the relative measurement technical error must be calculated. The formula to apply is the following:

$$\% \, TEM = \frac{TEM}{X} * 100$$

To obtain the relative measurement technical error, the intra-evaluator TEM is obtained as indicated above, and this result is divided by the average of the measurements taken from the same population with which the intra-evaluator TEM was calculated (X), and multiplied by 100 to obtain the percentage.

Next, an example is presented with the same data as those from the example given for the calculation of the intra-evaluator TEM. The following triceps skinfolds (mm) were measured in 10 elite senior women handball players (Table 4.2). It was observed in the previous calculation that the intra-evaluator TEM was 0.33 mm.

To know the relative TEM, the first thing to calculate is the average of the measurements taken from the same population. That is:

$$(9.9 + 9.3 + 8.6 + 8.7 + 11.6 + 10.6 + 10.3 + 10.5 + 11.7$$
$$+ 11.4 + 9.9 + 9.6 + 10.8 + 11.0 + 9.4 + 9.1 + 7.6 + 7.4 + 8.8$$
$$+ 8.2)/20 = 194.4/20 = 9.72$$

Next, you just have to divide the TEM/average and multiply the result by 100. In this case:

(0.33/9.72) * 100 = 3.4% of TEM relative to measuring the triceps skinfold in elite senior women handball players.

4.6.2 Validity

This is defined as the degree to which a measurement actually measures the characteristic it is intended to measure. In anthropometry, this is not a problem, as the variables are defined by themselves. Therefore, by following the ISAK protocol, the validity of the anthropometric assessment is taken for granted. However, the instruments should be validated, that is, it must be verified that the instruments measure what they intend to measure. Similarly, since the estimation of body composition is one of the most common applications after performing an anthropometric assessment, and all methods of estimating body composition are at least indirect, we should be concerned about the validity of these methods and/or the formulas applied in the estimation of body composition. More information on this is given in the specific topic of body composition.

4.6.3 Accuracy—Inter-rater TEM

Accuracy is defined as how close a value (measurement) is to the real value of the variable assessed. To find it, in the case of anthropometry, the final value obtained by the anthropometrist in a certain variable is compared with the final value of the variable obtained by a criterion anthropometrist (ISAK Level 4) or an instructor (ISAK Level 3).

To assess the accuracy of an anthropometrist as compared to the criterion, the formula for inter-rater TEM will be used. The formula to apply is the same as that for intra-rater TEM, but finding the differences between the value of a variable taken by the anthropometrist, whose accuracy is to be known, and the value of that same variable taken by the instructor or criterion anthropometrist. It is important to bear in mind that the measurements of both anthropometrists must be under the same conditions and with the same instruments, so that neither the biological variation of the subject, nor the variation between the measuring equipment, influence the result. In this way, it is recommended that the assessments of the subject studied by both anthropometrists, are as close as possible in time and without the subject having performed any behaviour that could influence the final result of the measurements. Thus, for the calculation of the absolute inter-rater TEM the following formula will be applied:

$$TEM = \sqrt{\frac{\Sigma d^2}{2n}}$$

where the TEM calculation will be carried out through the square root of the sum ($\sum$) of the squared differences of the final data from the measurement of the same variable on the same individual carried out by two different anthropometrists (d^2) divided by two times the number of subjects to whom that variable was measured (n), including the final value from each subject obtained by the anthropometrist, whose accuracy is to be known, and from an anthropometrist N3 or N4 as a reference for the real value of the measurement. It is important for the individual's biological variation to not influence the result obtained, that the two anthropometrists carry out the subject's measurements in the same evaluation session, following the previously specified measurement protocol.

Below is a numerical example of how to apply this. A novice anthropometrist and a criterion anthropometrist have measured the waist girth of 10 elite rhythmic gymnastics women in the same evaluation session, obtaining the following final values for each of them (the average in case of two measurements or the median in the case of three measurements according to the previously established protocol) (Table 4.6).

The steps to be taken for the inter-evaluator TEM calculation are:

1. Difference of the measurements made by the two anthropometrists for each of the subjects (Table 4.7).
2. The difference found for each of the subjects is squared (Table 4.8).

Table 4.6 Inter-evaluator TEM calculation: final data values of the measurements taken by two anthropometrists

Subject	1	2	3	4	5	6	7	8	9	10
Junior anthropometrist	59.9	54.2	56.8	60.1	58.8	61.5	55.6	57.4	56.7	60.0
Criterion anthropometrist	59.7	54.8	57.1	59.8	58.8	60.9	56.2	57.1	56.8	59.4

Table 4.7 Inter-evaluator TEM calculation: calculation of the differences between measurements taken by both anthropometrists

Subject	1	2	3	4	5	6	7	8	9	10
Diff anthropometrists	− 0.2	0.6	0.3	− 0.3	0.0	− 0.6	0.6	− 0.3	0.1	− 0.6

Table 4.8 Inter-evaluator TEM calculation: calculation of the square of the differences in the measurements taken by both anthropometrists

Subject	1	2	3	4	5	6	7	8	9	10
Diff ^{2}	0.04	0.36	0.09	0.09	0.00	0.36	0.36	0.09	0.01	0.36

Table 4.9 Inter-evaluator TEM calculation: sum of squared differences in the measurements taken by both anthropometrists

Total subjects	10
Sum Diff^2	$0.04 + 0.36 + 0.09 + 0.09 + 0.36 + 0.36 + 0.09 + 0.01 + 0.36 = 1.76$

3. All the squared differences of the 10 subjects are added up (Table 4.9).
4. The result is divided by 2 times the number of subjects: $1.76/2 * 10 = 0.088$.
5. The square root of the resulting value is taken: $\sqrt{0.088} = 0.296\,\text{cm}$.

However, the absolute inter-evaluator TEM does not allow the anthropometrist to know in which variables he/she is having a greater margin of error with respect to the criterion, as the absolute inter-evaluator TEM cannot be compared between the different variables, as they do not present similar values. Therefore, in order to know the percentage of error of the anthropometrist when taking a certain variable in a specific population, with respect to an anthropometrist N3 or N4, the relative measurement technical error must be calculated with the previously described formula.

Next, the relative inter-rater TEM will be calculated, continuing with the previous example. The waist girth of 10 elite rhythmic gymnastics women was measured (Table 4.6). It was obtained in the previous calculation that the inter-rater TEM was 0.296 cm.

To find the relative TEM, the first thing to calculate is the average of the measurements taken from the same population. This is:

$$(59.9 + 54.2 + 56.8 + 60.1 + 58.8 + 61.5 + 55.6 + 57.4 + 56.7 + 60 + 59.7 + 54.8 + 57.1 + 59.8 + 58.8 + 60.9 + 56.2 + 57.1 + 56.8 + 59.4)/20 = 1161.6/20 = 58.08\,\text{cm}.$$

Next, you just have to divide the TEM/average and multiply the result by 100. In this case:

(0.296/58.08) * 100 = 0.51% of relative TEM when measuring the waist girth in elite rhythmic gymnastics women.

Combining the concepts of intra-rater and inter-rater TEM, it can be determined if an anthropometrist is accurate (low intra-rater TEM) and precise (low inter-rater TEM). This is ideal and what is sought when any anthropometrist is trained. But it could also be the case that an anthropometrist is accurate but imprecise (low intra-rater TEM, but high inter-rater TEM), which could be attributable to a systematic error in the measurement. Under these circumstances, the anthropometrist will be able to analyse the change in their subjects, but not compare their values with any reference, as they are taking measurements differently. It could also be the case that the anthropometrist is inaccurate but precise (high intra-rater TEM and low inter-rater TEM), attributable to a random error in the measurement, although this is highly unlikely to happen, as it would indicate that the reported value resembles the value of the criterion anthropometrist with which the comparison was made by pure chance. Lastly, it could be that the anthropometrist is inaccurate and imprecise (high intra- and inter-rater TEM), due to the anthropometrist making systematic and random errors in the measurement. In this last case, the results or the changes found by this anthropometrist, or the measurements made with a reference population, could not be compared.

4.6.4 Probability of Success—Confidence Intervals

When an anthropometrist is monitoring the anthropometric changes of a subject over time, they can affirm that the changes that have occurred have been significant, have a tendency to change or do not have a tendency to change. For this, confidence intervals must be calculated. This statistical analysis can also be used to discover if a subject or population is significantly different or not to a reference subject or population, although confidence intervals are applied in this context on fewer occasions.

To be able to address this concept, it is necessary to start from the fact that when an anthropometrist makes a measurement, the value they obtain is not exact, as it is influenced by a contaminating factor due to their error as an anthropometrist. Thus, following the logic of the Gaussian bell, and taking the intra-rater TEM

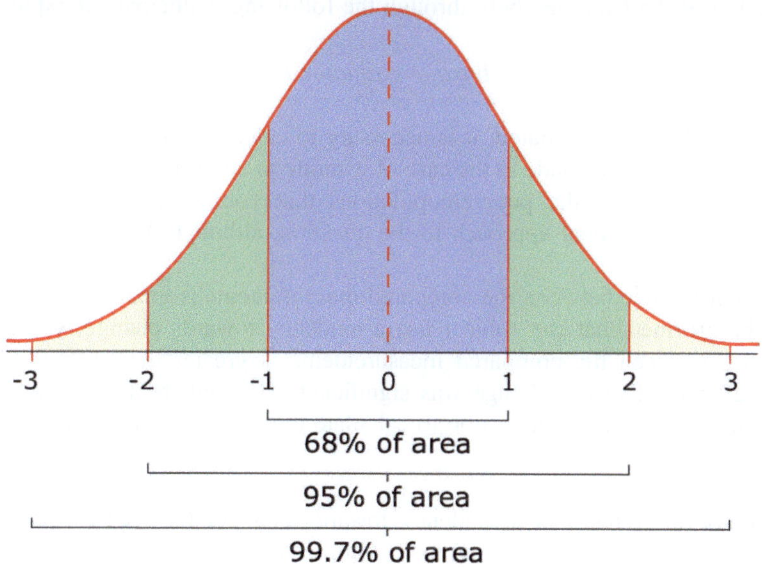

Fig. 4.1 Confidence intervals in a Gaussian distribution bell

for that variable as the standard deviation, three limits can be established in the confidence intervals between which the possible values of the measurement made to a subject can be found (Fig. 4.1).

Applying this concept, there can be a 68% certainty (68% confidence interval) that the value of a subject's measurement is found within the range of the measured value ± 1 * intra-rater TEM; at 95% (95% confidence interval) in the range of the measured value ± 2 * intra-evaluator TEM, and at 99.7% (confidence interval at 99%) in the range of the measured value ± 3 * intra-evaluator TEM. Thus, for example, if the 8 skinfold sum for a subject is 80 mm and the intra-evaluator TEM of the anthropometrist for the 8 skinfold sum in that population is 1 mm, it can be affirmed that at 68%, the value of the measured variable could oscillate between 79 and 81 mm; at 95% that the value of the measured variable could oscillate between 78 and 82 and at 99% that the value of the measured variable could oscillate between 77 and 83.

To compare the measurements made to two subjects with similar characteristics or the changes of a subject by comparing two measurements, to discover if the observed change is significant, is only a tendency towards change, or could be due to the assumed error in the measurement, this same logic of the Gaussian bell distribution will be followed by calculating the limits of the confidence interval for the detection of change based on the *standard error of difference* (SED). Therefore, the first thing we need to do is to address the concept of the SED, as it will be the error that is taken into consideration as a unit of the standard deviation in the application of the Gaussian bell, through the following mathematical expression:

$$SED = Intra - evaluator\, TEM * \sqrt{2}$$

Once the SED is calculated, it is necessary to calculate the difference between the two measurements made in the case of wanting to analyse a change, or between the measurements of the people/populations that you want to compare in the case of a cross-sectional approach to the question, although this approach is less common.

If the difference between the compared measurements is greater than the SED, it can be affirmed that the subject has a tendency towards change, while if the difference between the compared measurements is greater than 1.96 * SED, it can be affirmed that the change was significant. This will be translated into the following mathematical expression to calculate the following confidence intervals (CI):

> To discover if there is a tendency towards change: 68% CI = (Difference between measurements + SED) to (Difference between measurements − SED).
> To discover if the change is significant: 95% CI = (Difference between measurements + 1.96 * SED) to (Difference between measurements − 1.96 * SED).

If within the range of values reported by these equations you have to pass through "0" to move from one number to another, in other words, if the limits shown are a positive number and a negative number, it cannot be affirmed that there is a tendency towards change for the calculation of the 68% CI, or that the change is significant for the calculation of the 95% CI. In turn, if the reported values are two positive numbers or two negative numbers, to go from one to the other, there will be no need to pass through "0". Then, it can be affirmed that there is a tendency for change in the calculation of the 68% CI or that the change is significant for the calculation of the 95% CI. This is important, as it provides certainty to how the change of a particular subject is occurring, in order to make the relevant adjustments in the nutritional or training plan of that individual, to move in the direction of the objective set. In this sense, when applying a training programme or a nutritional plan, if the subject shows results contrary to those sought, which we will be able to know thanks to the application of the CIs, the other factors must be reviewed.

Below is a practical example of the application of what explained above. A subject is measured before and after a period of high intensity training with caloric restriction. It is found that the 8 skinfold sum of the subject before starting the measurement was 80 and after eight weeks of training it is 75 mm. The TEM intra-evaluator of the anthropometrist for the 8 skinfold sum is 1 mm. The first thing to calculate is the SED, which is equal to $1 * \sqrt{2} = 1.41$ mm.

Next, we have to calculate the difference between both measurements. In this case, $80 - 75 = 5$ mm.

We continue by calculating the 68% CI to find if there is a tendency for change. Therefore, 5 + 1.41 to 5 − 1.41 = 6.41 to 3.59. As they are two positive numbers, and to go from one to the other there is no need to pass through "0", it can be affirmed that at least there is a tendency for change.

Finally, we are going to calculate the 95% CI to see if the change is significant. Therefore, 5 + 1.96 * 1.41 to 5 − 1.96 * 1.41 = 5 + 2.80 to 5 − 2.8 = 7.76 to 2.24. As they are two positive numbers, and to go from one to the other there is no need to pass through "0", it can be affirmed that the change is significant.

In conclusion, our subject has significantly decreased his/her 8 skinfold sum with the work performed, and we can affirm this with total certainty.

One last issue to consider is that in case a comparison does not show a tendency to be significant, it is not necessary to see if the change is significant as it will not be; while, if a change is significant, it is not necessary to analyse if it has a tendency to be so as it will be.

In summary, everything discussed in this chapter is necessary for:

- Minimising the errors made when conducting an anthropometric assessment.
- Indicating the degree of precision of an anthropometrist.
- Indicating the accuracy of an anthropometrist.
- When several anthropometrists take a measurement, to determine the inter-evaluator TEM.
- Indicate the intra-evaluator and inter-evaluator TEM of a study, as an indicator of the quality of the measurement.
- Indicate the results with an appropriate confidence interval.
- Demonstrate real changes in a specific measurement.

4.7 Questionnaire

1. One of the most common errors in anthropometric measurements is:
   (a) Lack of standardisation in measurements.
   (b) Taking measurements on the right side.
   (c) Marking the points to be measured before starting the measurement.
   (d) Taking the skinfold with the fingers tangent just before the cross.
2. Whenever possible, it is recommended to work in a troika when performing anthropometric measurements, which means:
   (a) That only the anthropometrist and the subject being assessed will participate in it.
   (b) The more people there are in the measurement room, the better, as long as they do not disturb the anthropometrist.
   (c) The anthropometrist, the subject to be measured and the recorder/assistant will participate in the measurements.
   (d) None of the above.

3. Regarding the assistant's role in the measurements:
   (a) They will repeat the measurement indicated by the anthropometrist to ensure that the notation was correct.
   (b) They can assist the anthropometrist in some measurements, such as in the case of girths.
   (c) They can indicate to the anthropometrist the next measurement that should be taken next.
   (d) All of the above are true.
4. The performance of several measurements of each variable in an anthropometric assessment:
   (a) Only serves to increase the chances of making a mistake.
   (b) It is within the ISAK protocols and serves to minimise random error.
   (c) The first and second measurement of the same variable are performed consecutively.
   (d) The third measurement is always optional, as the protocol does not specify when it should be used.
5. When the error made between the first and second measurement of a skinfold is greater than 5%:
   (a) The final value taken is the first one.
   (b) The final value taken is the average of the values.
   (c) A third measurement is made and the final value taken is the median.
   (d) A third measurement is made and the final value taken is the average of the three.
6. Among the possible individual factors that can affect the measurement, the following is not included:
   (a) The time at which the measurement is taken.
   (b) The practice of exercise close to the measurement time.
   (c) The thickness or elasticity of the skin.
   (d) The verification of the equipment.
7. Indicate the true answer in relation to common errors in data collection and recording:
   (a) Auditory error is one of the most common.
   (b) If the assistant is unfamiliar with the anthropometric technique, an identification error of the measurement can occur.
   (c) Depending on the type of instrumentation used, the anthropometrist can make a reading error if they are not familiar.
   (d) All are true.
8. The proximity of a measurement to the real value of the variable assessed, is called:
   (a) Precision.
   (b) Accuracy.
   (c) Reliability.
   (d) Validity.

9. Given a triceps skinfold of 9.3 mm and knowing that the TEM of the anthropometrist is 0.3, what would be the values of the 95% confidence interval?
   (a) 8.7 and 9.9.
   (b) 9.0 and 9.6.
   (c) 8.4 and 10.2.
   (d) With this data, it cannot be calculated.
10. Regarding the standard error of the difference (SED):
   (a) If the range set for the 68% confidence interval passes through the value "0", there is a tendency towards change.
   (b) If the range set for the 95% confidence interval passes through the value "0", there are significant differences.
   (c) The SED is not useful for knowing if there is a tendency to change or a significant change.
   (d) All are false.

Answers

1.a 2.c 3.d 4.b 5.c 6.d 7.d 8.b 9.a 10.d

Bibliography

Carter, J. E. L., & Ackland, T. (1994). *Kinanthropometry in aquatic sports. A study of world class athletes*. Human Kinetics.

Clarys, J. P., Martin, A. D., Drinkwater, D. T., & Marfell-Jones, M. J. (1987). The skinfold: Myth and reality. *Journal of Sports Sciences, 5*, 3–33.

Esparza-Ros, F., Vaquero-Cristóbal, R., & Marfell-Jones, M. (2019). *International protocol for anthropometric assessment*. International Society for the Advancement of Kinanthropometry.

Lampl, M. (1992). Further observations on diurnal variation in standing height. *Annals of Human Biology, 19*, 87–90.

Norton, K., & Olds, T. (1996). *Anthropometrica*. University of New South Wales Press.

Analysis of Body Composition Through Anthropometric Assessment

5

Abstract

This chapter addresses the importance of evaluating body composition, especially in the sports and health fields. Various models for estimating body composition are presented, highlighting the tissue model as one of the most utilized, as it allows differentiating between specific tissues such as adipose, bone, and muscle. The text also points out a common terminological error in the field of body composition, where the term 'fat mass' is generically used, although in reality other components such as lipid mass or adipose tissue are being estimated. This leads to confusion and to considering different concepts as synonyms when they are not. Following this, the chapter analyses different methods for estimating body composition, such as dual-energy X-ray absorptiometry (DXA or DEXA), hydrodensitometry or hydrostatic weighing (UWW), air displacement plethysmography (ADP), electrical bioimpedance or anthropometry, with an analysis conducted on their advantages and disadvantages. Subsequently, the estimation of body composition from anthropometry as an indirect or double indirect method, depending on how it is approached, is addressed. Bicompartmental, tetracompartmental, and pentacompartmental models are detailed for estimating body composition through anthropometric measurements, providing the equations recommended for use in each context. Finally, the use of the sum of skinfolds and corrected girths as alternatives for evaluating body composition is discussed, highlighting their usefulness in relation to adiposity and muscle development.

Keywords

Fat mass • Lipid mass • Adipose tissue • Muscle mass • Anthropometry • Bioimpedance • X-ray densitometry • Sum of skinfolds • Corrected girths

© The Author(s), under exclusive license to Springer Nature Switzerland AG 2025

F. Esparza-Ros and R. Vaquero-Cristóbal, *Anthropometry*,
https://doi.org/10.1007/978-3-031-77535-2_5

5.1 Introduction

Body composition, proportionality, and somatotype are the three main areas of application of anthropometry. The three areas present some advantages and disadvantages as will be observed in the specific topics, so that it is necessary to know all three, as they are complementary in the interpretation of anthropometry through its derived variables.

Starting with body composition, this is perhaps the most well-known concept when performing an anthropometric assessment. It allows for the estimation of both plastic components, that is, adipose and muscle, as well as structural components, among which the bone component stands out, so its analysis has been a recurring topic of study in the sports field and also in the health field.

Body composition estimation is defined as the method that allows estimating the body mass fractionally, and relating the derived components with the environment and the habits of the subject. It is important to start by knowing that, when performing an exact assessment of the body composition of a subject, it cannot be calculated, because to calculate body composition, it is necessary to perform a direct method and the only direct method is dissection, which is not applicable to living subjects. Therefore, when we assess body composition, what we are really doing is estimating it. As a consequence of the above, all methods used for the assessment of body composition have a margin of error, even those that have been classically considered as reference methods, such as dual-energy X-ray absorptiometry (DEXA or DXA).

5.2 Models for the Estimation of Body Composition

Body composition estimation can be performed with different models. The currently known models are:

- Model 1: Chemical elements/atoms. This model divides the body based on the chemical elements that compose it. Thus, according to this approach, the body is composed of 64% oxygen, 18.5% carbon, 9.5% hydrogen, 3.2% nitrogen, 1.5% calcium, 1% phosphorus and 2.3% other components. This model is not used in the field of body composition estimation.
- Model 2: Molecular. This model divides the body into molecules based on the micro and macronutrients that compose it, with the molecules being the following: lipids (about 15%), proteins (about 18%), carbohydrates (about 1%), minerals (about 6%), and water (about 60%). In this model, fat mass is not estimated, what is estimated is lipid content, resulting in two components: lipid mass and lipid-free mass. However, it is classically indicated that with this model, fat mass is estimated. In this model, body composition has been traditionally addressed with techniques such as hydrodensitometry; air displacement plethysmography; bioelectrical impedance; DXA; or most of the formulas for estimating "fat" mass with anthropometry, except for the Kerr formula.

In this model, the following alternatives can be chosen:
- Two-compartment model: lipid mass and lipid-free mass.

- Model 3: Cellular. From the perspective of this model, the body is broken down according to the cells that compose it, differentiating between: fat (about 18%), extracellular solids (about 9%), intracellular solids (about 12%), intracellular fluids (about 34%), and extracellular fluids (about 27%). When a two-compartment approach is taken from this model, it comprises fat mass and fat-free mass. This model is not usually used in the approach to body composition.
- Model 4: Tissue. This is a model that allows addressing body composition by breaking down the body into tissues. It allows differentiating between adipose tissue (about 25%), bone tissue (about 10%), skeletal muscle tissue (about 33%), and non-skeletal muscle tissue and soft tissues (residual tissue) (about 29%). This is one of the most used models in the approach to body composition from the field of sport, but also health, as the rest of the models estimate the lipid or fat mass and assume that the rest of the tissues are fat-free or lipid-free mass, assuming that changes in fat-free mass are due to changes in muscle mass, when this might not be true, as fat-free mass includes more tissues than muscle mass itself, so changes cannot be solely attributed to this tissue. However, from this tissue model, skeletal muscle tissue can be tracked, analysing its change in isolation, without it being influenced a priori by changes in other components.

  This makes it a very advantageous model from the point of view of the sports field due to its relationship with sports performance, but also in the field of health due to its relationship with certain diseases such as sarcopenia, so the use of this model is necessary when the intention is to find the muscle mass.

  In this model, the following approach alternatives are usually chosen:
  - Four-compartment model: adipose tissue, skeletal muscle, bone and residual.
  - Five-compartment model: adipose tissue, bone, skeletal muscle, residual and skin.

  This approach model has been used by anthropometry, when addressing body composition with Kerr's 5-component model for "fat" and with different body composition formulas for the rest of the components. Also by some other methods based on image analysis, such as magnetic resonance (MR), Computed Axial Tomography (CAT) or ultrasound.
- Model 5: Body segments. This model allows addressing body composition through different body segments. Thus, from this model, the estimation of the mass of each of the upper and lower limbs, the trunk, and the head has traditionally been addressed. However, this method is not usually used, as it does not allow differentiating between the most predominant tissues in each of these segments or their change, which limits its application in the field of sport and health.

It is important to conclude this description of the different approach models knowing that, although most body composition estimation models address it from model 2 (molecular) or model 4 (tissue), leading to the estimation of lipid mass and adipose tissue, respectively, as representatives of the amount of adiposity, in the field of body composition estimation a significant terminological error has traditionally been made. Thus, regardless of the model used, all techniques talk about the estimation of fat mass, when it is not really the case. This is because to estimate fat mass, one would have to address it from model 3 (cellular), which is not done. Not surprisingly, most of these software discuss fat mass when they are not estimating it, but rather they estimate lipid mass or adipose tissue depending on the approach model they use. This has led to the use of synonymous concepts when they are not, as addressed below.

5.3 Lipid Mass, Fat Mass or Adipose Tissue? A Relevant Consideration

One of the main drawbacks in the field of body composition estimation is the indiscriminate use of the terms adipose tissue, fat mass, and lipid mass.

The term adipose tissue refers to the mass of the adipocytes (Fig. 5.1). It is composed of fat mass up to 90%, but also by water and minerals by 10%. Therefore, when analysing adipose tissue, that percentage of water and minerals is being included.

In turn, fat mass is 83% lipids and 16% glycerol (Fig. 5.2).

Therefore, lipid mass is a subcomponent of fat mass, and fat mass a subcomponent of adipose tissue, so the term "fat mass" cannot be used synonymously with "adipose mass/adipose tissue" or "lipid mass".

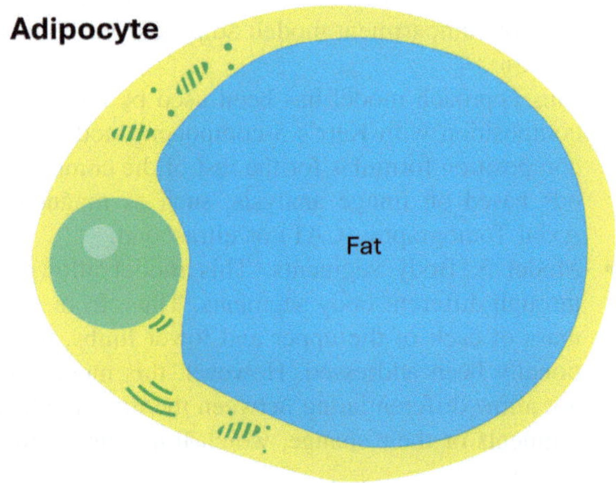

Fig. 5.1 Composition of the adipocyte

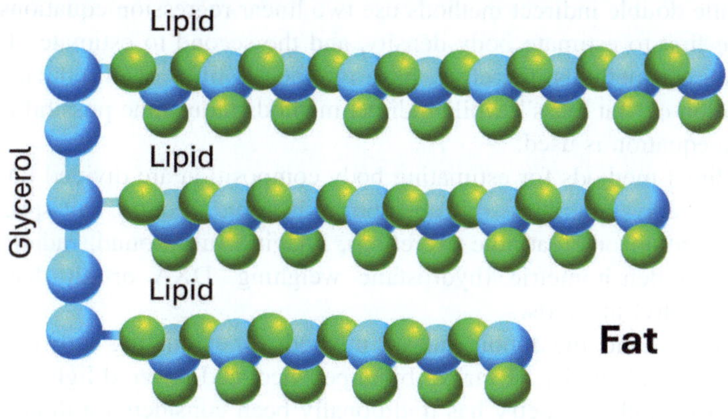

Fig. 5.2 Composition of fat (triglyceride)

To understand the implications of this, an example is presented below. A woman with body mass of 70 kg is assessed, resulting in 30% adipose tissue. This corresponds to 21 kg of adipose tissue. Taking into account that 90% of this is fat mass, if fat mass were estimated instead of adipose tissue, the result would be 21 kg * 0.90 = 18.9 kg (18.9/70 = 27.00% of fat mass). Considering that in turn, lipid mass is 83% fat mass, if lipid mass is estimated instead of fat mass, the result would be 18.9 kg * 0.83 = 15.69 kg (15.69/70 = 22.41% of lipid mass). Therefore, if the term "fat mass" is erroneously used to indistinctly refer to these concepts, depending on the approach chosen, a "fat mass" percentage of 30, 27 or 22.41% will be found, along with a kg estimate of "fat mass" of 21, 18.9 or 15.69 kg, with the original data actually being the same. Therefore, it is essential to know how adiposity is being addressed when assessing a subject and whether lipid mass, fat mass, or adipose tissue is truly being estimated.

5.4 Most Commonly Used Methods for Estimating Body Composition

The direct method for calculating body composition is cadaver dissection. Between the years 1979 and 1984, a study was carried out at the University of Brussels, under the direction of Prof. William Ross, which served as a doctoral thesis for various experts in anthropometry. This study included 25 cadavers, 12 men and 13 women, aged between 55 and 94 years, who underwent an exhaustive dissection, and whose results have been used as a reference for the validation of the rest of the indirect and double indirect methods of estimating body composition and the different formulas used.

In this sense, indirect methods are known as those that calculate body density, after which a linear regression equation or an algorithm is used to estimate "fat mass", while double indirect methods use two linear regression equations or algorithms, the first to estimate body density, and the second to estimate "fat mass". Double indirect methods, therefore, have two possibilities of introducing error in the estimation of "fat mass", while indirect methods reduce the possibility of error as a single equation is used.

The indirect methods for estimating body composition are divided into physicochemical (plethysmography, gas absorption, isotopic dilution, ray spectrometry, neutron activation or creatinine excretion), imaging (ultrasound, radiology, CAT or MR), and densitometric (hydrostatic weighing, DXA or air displacement plethysmography) methods.

On the other hand, the double indirect methods for estimating body composition are electrical conductivity, electrical bioimpedance, and infrared light reactance.

On its part, anthropometry has traditionally been considered a double indirect method, which is true in most cases. However, if body composition is addressed with this method, through the use of the five-component mathematical method of Kerr, anthropometry becomes an indirect method for estimating body composition. The most commonly used methods for estimating body composition are as follows:

5.4.1 Dual-Energy X-ray Densitometry (DXA or DEXA)

This is an indirect method for estimating body composition. Dual-energy X-ray densitometry aims to estimate body composition from model 2 (molecular), and differentiates between: lipid mass, lean mass, and bone mineral content. Included within the densitometric techniques, this method uses low-exposure X-rays to detect the energy of photons, to differentiate between bone mineral content and the rest of the molecules, at the same time that it is able to differentiate within them, between lipids and the rest of the molecules.

Its main advantage is that it is a precise method, being considered by many as the gold standard for estimating bone mineral content. Regarding the disadvantages, it assumes that the amount of adiposity on the bone is proportional to the existing adiposity on the non-bone tissue, with this being a significant disadvantage in the estimation of adiposity. Thus, its use as a gold standard in the assessment of fat mass has been highly questioned, being considered rather a reference method, as it is the most commonly method used for this purpose. Another of its handicaps in this same line is that it claims to estimate fat mass in its reports, when in reality what it estimates is lipid mass.

Furthermore, it assumes that the degree of hydration of muscle mass is constant, which is a disadvantage for estimating lean mass. As a consequence of this, there is scientific consensus that it cannot be considered the gold standard in the estimation of muscle mass, with the gold standard for the determination of this tissue being MR.

The other limitations are that it requires great precision and training of the evaluators to adjust the body areas, as this process must be done manually. In addition, the software cannot be updated, as it changes the database and the values it reports. If it were necessary to compare the values of different software programs or different versions of the same software, it is necessary to extract the raw data without comparing it with the software population to avoid this error. Finally, another problem with this technique is that it is a high-cost device and not portable.

5.4.2 Hydrodensitometry or Underwater Weighing (UWW)

This indirect method studies body composition from model 2 (molecular), allowing for the differentiation between lipid mass and lipid-free mass. It is based on Archimedes' principle by which a body totally or partially submerged in a fluid at rest, experiences an upward thrust equal to the mass of the displaced fluid. This method basically consists of comparing a person's normal mass outside of water, with their mass when submerged, analysing the water displaced by the body when it is completely submerged to measure the body volume after estimating the residual lung volume, using the former to calculate body density. With this body density it estimates the lipid mass.

Its main advantage is the precision in the measurement, but among its disadvantages we find the cost of the system, which is not portable, and also requiring a long measurement time, aside from it being uncomfortable for the subject. It is not an easy technique to use, because to achieve the highest degree of accuracy, it needs a precise measurement of body mass outside and inside the water, the water temperature, and the residual lung volume, at the same time that it requires a considerable amount of time, space, equipment, and experience from the researchers.

5.4.3 Air Displacement Plethysmography (ADP)

It is an indirect method that estimates body composition based on model 2 (molecular), which allows differentiating between lipid mass and lipid-free mass. This method analyses the volume of air displaced in a closed fibreglass chamber in which the subject is seated, using computerised pressure and volume sensors to obtain body density, to then estimate the lipid mass. It requires a plethysmograph that is commercially named "BOD POD". Its main advantages are the measurement time and ease of use, while among the disadvantages we find the cost of the device, that it is not a portable system and the error that occurs in the estimation of the residual lung volume, even when this test is done by performing a forced exhalation.

5.4.4 Bioelectrical Impedance Analysis (BIA)

This double indirect method estimates body composition based on model 2 (molecular), allowing for the differentiation between lipid mass and lipid-free mass. In the best case, it also includes water as a third component.

This technique consists of predicting body composition based on the electrical conducting properties of the body. Bioelectrical impedance measures the resistance or opposition to the flow of current, taking advantage of the electrolytes present in body water being excellent conductors of electrical current. It measures electrical properties: impedance, resistance, reactance, and phase angle. For this, it transmits a very low power electrical current through the body and calculates the time it takes for this current to travel through it, estimating the body density, and after this, the lipid mass.

When the total volume of water is large, the current flows more easily through the body and with less resistance. Therefore, individuals with a large amount of fat-free mass or total water volume present less resistance to the current. On the contrary, individuals with large amounts of body fat present more resistance to the flow of the current because the water content in adipose tissue is poor.

Bearing this in mind, bioelectrical impedance assumes that the muscle, having a greater amount of water, conducts electricity more quickly than fat; that fat conducts electricity poorly and that all muscles always have the same degree of hydration, which is a mistake. Some other drawbacks of this technique are that all factors that affect hydration affect the validity of the method (liquid intake, sports practice, menstrual cycle, medication, etc.), and that it is less valid the fewer electrodes the instrument has, increasing the price of the bioimpedance scale with the inclusion of more electrodes. The main advantages are the speed in the measurement, it is not an invasive method, and it is affordable from the start, although it depends on the instrument with which it is carried out, as the bioimpedance scales with more than six channels command higher prices. Other advantages are the low intra and inter observer variability they may have, it does not require specialised personnel for the assessment, it does not require collaboration from the patient, and that it is a portable method, although the most valid bioimpedance scales are heavier, which makes their transport somewhat more difficult.

To try to minimise the error in the measurement with electrical impedance, some criteria have been defined for the standardisation of the measurement. With their compliance, bioimpedance can be considered an accurate and precise method. Thus, bioimpedance should be performed:

- First thing in the morning on an empty stomach.
- Do not eat or drink 4 h before.
- Do not perform strenuous exercise in the 12 h prior.
- Urinate 30 min before.
- Do not take diuretics 7 days before.
- Do not perform it in the luteal phase as it is a phase of the menstrual cycle in which a large amount of fluid is retained.

- Remove metals such as watches, rings, piercings, etc.
- A urine colour test should be included to ensure normal hydration status when performing the test.

As a result of these criteria, the bioelectrical impedance method is difficult to apply correctly in a clinic. If these criteria are not followed, the subject's hydration will be affected, significantly influencing the validity of the measurement.

5.4.5 Anthropometry

It is a valid technique as long as a standardised measurement protocol is followed, among which we undoubtedly find that the one most widely disseminated worldwide is the protocol by the International Society for the Advancement of Kinanthropometry (ISAK). Regarding the advantages of this method, it is not invasive, it is affordable, it allows assessment in different contexts, and provides more results than the single study of body composition. The main disadvantage is that specific training is needed by the measurer to be able to take the measurements accurately and reliably. In addition, it is a complex model, as it can be considered a double indirect method if the lipid mass is addressed based on model 2 (molecular), or indirect if the adipose tissue is addressed based on model 4 (tissue). More specifically, with anthropometry, body composition can be addressed in the following manner:

- Bicompartmental model: It allows differentiating between lipid mass and lipid-free mass. In this model, anthropometry is used to take a series of measurements of different skinfolds, which are used to estimate body density, after which the lipid mass can be estimated. It is therefore an indirect double model that addresses body composition based on model 2 (molecular). Most of the equations used in anthropometry are under the umbrella of this model, with more than 100 equations for the estimation of lipid mass, where each has been validated in a specific context and with a specific population and can only and should be applied in that same context. In fact, recent studies have shown that the formulas used to estimate lipid mass are not interchangeable, even when applied in the same population in which they were validated, as there are significant differences between all the formulas for the estimation of lipid mass. Within these equations, perhaps the most well-known are the equations by Faulkner (1968), Durnin and Womersley (1975), Jackson and Pollock (1978), Carter (1982) or Withers (1987). The main drawback of the approach to body composition with anthropometry from this perspective is that it is an indirect double method, in which the error of two linear regression equations accumulate, so that it cannot be applied to the equations in a different context in which they were validated, and that the results reported by the different equations are not comparable. Not surprisingly, this leads to, in the same individual, according to the chosen formula, a variation of up to 10% in lipid mass, incorrectly called fat mass.

- Four-compartment model: the use of anthropometry based on this model has traditionally estimated the lipid component based on model 2 (molecular), and the rest of the components from model 4 (tissue), assuming that lipid mass is the same as adipose tissue. As has been seen previously, this is not correct. To estimate the lipid mass from this model, a series of skinfolds are taken, through which body density is estimated, as well as the lipid mass. But it also relies on the measurement of other anthropometric measurements (girths and breadths) to, through linear regression equations, estimate the muscle-skeletal, bone, and residual tissue. Therefore, it is an indirect double method for lipid mass and indirect for the rest of the masses, mixing models and assuming that lipid mass and adipose tissue are the same, with this assumption being its main drawback.

  By addressing lipid mass through the use of the molecular model, and the rest of the components through the tissue model, the estimation of the four components separately provides a very large margin of error in relation to total body mass.

  Another alternative is to assume that the result of total body mass minus the mass of the other three components gives rise to the fourth component. However, care must be taken when doing this, as in this last component, not only what corresponds to it is included, but the error derived from the estimation of the three previous compartments also accumulates. This is especially serious when the component that is estimated as the remainder to the others is the muscular component, as observed in the case of Rose and Guimarães' strategy, which led to it receiving a large number of criticisms for overestimating muscle mass in women and for estimating residual mass with a constant.

  Thus, without being an idyllic option, it is better to drag this error from the estimation of the different components to the residual component, as it has a lesser application in the sports or health fields. In this way, the skeletal muscle mass could be estimated with Lee's formula (2000) in all populations, which is not entirely correct, as it should not be used in populations different from those in which it was validated, although there is no better alternative that does not include a large amount of anthropometric variables to measure; and the bone mass with Rocha's formula (1978) in most of the population, except in the older population, where it would be advisable to use Martin's formula (1991) and estimate the result of subtracting the other three components from the total body mass, as the residual mass.

  Finally, to avoid the problem of mixing models in the approach to body composition from a tetracompartmental perspective, a proposal is made to address the component related to adiposity not from an estimation of the lipid mass (model 2: molecular), but from an estimation of the adipose tissue, to address all components based on model 4 (tissue), in order to avoid mixing models. Therefore, a possible solution would be to estimate the adipose tissue with Kerr's formula

(1991). Moreover, this formula comes from a mathematical model, so it is an indirect method, instead of double indirect one.

In this way and in summary, the tetracompartmental approach proposal would be: adipose tissue with Kerr's formula (1991); skeletal muscle tissue with Lee's formula (2000); bone tissue with Rocha's formula (1978) for all populations and Martin's formula (1991) for older population; and residual tissue as the result of subtracting the other three components from the total body mass.

- Pentacompartmental model: it is known as the five components model of Kerr (1991). This model is based on the taking of a series of anthropometric measurements (basic measurements, skinfolds, girths, and breadths and depths) at previously marked anthropometric points for the estimation of the masses with the use of the tissue model (model 4).

  It is considered the most reliable model in the field of anthropometry due to different aspects. Firstly, it is a mathematical model that does not need to estimate body density, so it is an indirect model in the estimation of the adipose component, not double indirect as we find when lipid mass is estimated with the rest of the models. Another great advantage of this method is that it was directly validated with the data obtained through cadaver dissection, which is the gold standard for measuring body composition. Another of its main advantages is that it does not estimate any of the components as the result of subtracting the other components from the total body mass of the individual. In other words, it has its own equation for the estimation of each of the components. When the sum of the estimated masses of each of the components has been compared with the total body mass of the subject, it has been found that the difference is in most cases ± 1 kg. It is, therefore, a very valid and precise method. Its main disadvantage is the measurement time required due to the number of variables included in the formulas that compose it, some of which can be somewhat invasive if care is not taken when taking them.

Due to all the existing methods to estimate body composition and the differences between them in addressing this topic, the different scientific studies that have analysed the existing differences in the comparison of the different methods used for the estimation of body composition have concluded that the methods are not comparable. That is, the estimation values of body composition found by DXA, hydrostatic weighing, air displacement plethysmography, anthropometry, or bioimpedance, among others, cannot be compared. Moreover, if the instrument, the equation or the software used are changed, even when always using the same method, the results will also not comparable. However, the different methods are reliable, and therefore, the method, the instrument, and the formulas or software used must be maintained if a longitudinal study is carried out, or if the intention is to compare subjects in a reliable way. In addition, the most affordable methods, that is, anthropometry and bioelectrical impedance, present validity problems in most of their formulas. This results in the bioelectrical impedance being considered a valid method to analyse populations, but not to analyse subjects individually. On the other hand, in anthropometry, it is common for the formulas to be used regardless of the context in which they were validated, which reduces their validity.

In conclusion, all methods of estimating body composition have advantages and disadvantages. There seems to be some consensus that DXA could be the best method for globally estimating body composition, without it being an ideal method. However, this can only be done with guarantees if there is a standardisation of the time of day at which the measurement is taken, the use of supplements, the intake of food and liquids, the practice of exercise, and the glycogen content in the liver and muscles. In the event of not being able to comply with these standardised considerations regarding the subject's condition, the alternative would be to use anthropometry, as this method is least affected by non-compliance with standard conditions by the individuals to be analysed.

5.5 Analysis of Body Composition from Anthropometry

As a result of the above, in the case of wanting to estimate body composition by means of anthropometry, a five-component approach (pentacompartmental model) with the equations of Kerr (1991) is recommended. These are:

- Adipose component: Kerr (1991). The measurement of the triceps, subscapular, supraspinal, abdominal, thigh and calf skinfolds is necessary.

$$\text{1st } \Sigma\ 6 \text{ skinfolds} = \text{Triceps skinfold (mm)} + \text{Subscapular skinfold (mm)} + \text{Supraspinal skinfold (mm)} + \text{Abdominal skinfold (mm)} + \text{Thigh skinfold (mm)} + \text{Calf skinfold (mm)}$$

$$\text{2nd Z adiposity} = [\Sigma 6 \text{ skinfolds} * (170.18/\text{Stretch stature (cm)}) - 116.41]/34.79.$$

where:
- 170.18 = mode of the *Phantom* method for Stretch stature (cm).
- 116.41 = sum of the mode of the skinfolds of the *Phantom* method (mm).
- 34.79 = sum of the standard deviations for the skinfolds of the *Phantom* method (mm).

$$\text{3rd Adipose mass(kg)} = \left[(\text{Z adiposity} * 5.85) + 25.6\right] / (170.18/\text{Stretch stature (cm)})^3$$

Where:

- 5.85 = standard deviation of the *Phantom* method for the adipose mass (kg).
- 25.6 = mode of the *Phantom* method for the adipose mass (kg).
- 170.18 = mode of the *Phantom* method for stretch stature (cm).

• Muscular component: Kerr (1991). It is necessary to measure the arm relaxed, forearm, chest, thigh middle, and calf girths, and the triceps, subscapular, thigh, and calf skinfolds.

$$\begin{aligned}\text{1st } \Sigma \text{ Girths} = {} & \text{Corrected arm girth (cm)} + \text{Forearm girth (cm)} \\ & + \text{Corrected thigh girth (cm)} + \text{Corrected calf girth (cm)} \\ & + \text{Corrected chest girth (cm)}\end{aligned}$$

where:

- Corrected arm girth = Arm relaxed girth (cm) − π * triceps skinfold (cm).
- Corrected thigh girth = Thigh middle girth (cm) − π * thigh skinfold (cm).
- Corrected calf girth = Calf girth (cm) − π * calf skinfold (cm).
- Corrected chest girth = Chest girth (cm) − π * subscapular skinfold (cm).

$$\begin{aligned}\text{2nd Z muscle mass} = {} & [(\Sigma \text{ Girths} * (170.18 \\ & /\text{Stretch stature (cm)} \\ & - 207.21/13.74)]\end{aligned}$$

where:

- 170.18 = mode of the *Phantom* method for stretch stature (cm).
- 207.21 = sum of the mode of corrected arm girth + Forearm girth + Corrected thigh girth + Corrected calf girth + Corrected chest girth of the *Phantom* method (cm).
- 13.74 = sum of the standard deviations for Corrected arm girth + Forearm girth + Corrected thigh girth + Corrected calf girth + Corrected chest girth of the *Phantom* method (cm).

$$\begin{aligned}\text{3rd Muscle mass (kg)} = {} & [(\text{Z muscle mass} * 5.4) + 24.5] \\ & /(170.18/\text{Stretch stature (cm)})^3\end{aligned}$$

where:

- 5.45 = standard deviation of the *Phantom* method for muscle mass (kg).
- 24.5 = mode of the *Phantom* method for muscle mass (kg).

• Bone component: Kerr (1991). It is necessary to measure the head girth and the biacromial, biiliocristal, humerus and femur breadths. It should be taken into account that the bone masses of the head and body are calculated independently.

$$\text{1st Z Head} = (\text{Head girth (cm)} - 56.0)/1.44$$

where:
- 56.0 = mode of the *Phantom* method for head girth (cm).
- 1.44 = standard deviation of the *Phantom* method for head girth (cm).

$$\text{2nd H Head} = (\text{Z Head} * 0.18) + 1.20$$

where:
- 0.18 = standard deviation of the *Phantom* method for the bone mass of the head (kg).
- 1.20 = mode of the *Phantom* method for the bone mass of the head (kg).

$$\text{3rd } \Sigma \text{ Breadths} = (\text{Biacromial breadth (cm)} + \text{Biiliocristal breadth (cm)} + 2 * \text{Humerus breadth (cm)} + 2 * \text{Femur breadth (cm)})$$

$$\text{4th Z Body} = (\Sigma \text{ Breadths} * 170.18/\text{Stretch stature (cm)}) - 98.88/5.33$$

where:
- 170.18 = Mode of the *Phantom* method for stretch stature (cm).
- 98.88 = sum of the mode of Biacromial breadth + Biiliocristal breadth + 2 * Humerus breadth + 2 * Femur breadth of the *Phantom* method (cm).
- 13.74 = sum of the standard deviations for Biacromial breadth + Biiliocristal breadth + 2 * Humerus breadth + 2 * Femur breadth of the *Phantom* method (cm).

$$\text{5th H Body} = (\text{Z Body} * 1.34 + 6.70)/(170.18/\text{Stretch stature (cm)})^3$$

where:
- 1.34 = standard deviation of the *Phantom* method for the bone mass of the body (kg).
- 6.70 = mode of the *Phantom* method for the bone mass of the body (kg).
- 170.18 = mode of the *Phantom* method for stretch stature (cm).

$$\text{6th Total bone mass (kg)} = \text{H Body} + \text{H Head}$$

- Skin component: Kerr (1991). Body mass and stretch stature variables are needed.

$$\text{1st Body surface} = K_1 * \text{Body mass (kg)}^{0.425} * \text{Stretch stature (cm)}^{0.725}/10000$$

where:
- K_1 = body surface constant = 68.308 for men aged over 12 years, 73.704 for women aged over 12 years, and 70.691 for men and women under 12 years.

$$2\text{nd Skin mass (kg)} = \text{Body surface} * K_2 * 1.05$$

where:
- K_2 = skin thickness constant, 2.07 for men and 1.96 for women.
- 1.05 = skin density.

- Residual component: Kerr (1991). The measurement of the waist girth, the abdominal skinfold and the antero-posterior chest depth and transverse chest breadth and the sitting height are necessary.

$$\begin{aligned}1\text{st } \Sigma \text{ Residual} = {} & \text{Antero-posterior chest depth (cm)} \\ & + \text{Transverse chest breadth (cm)} \\ & + \text{Corrected waist girth (cm)}\end{aligned}$$

where:
- Corrected waist girth = waist girth (cm) − π * Abdominal skinfold (cm).

$$2\text{nd Z Residual} = \left[\Sigma \text{ Residual} * (89.92/\text{Sitting height (cm)}) - 109.35\right]/7.08$$

where:
- 89.92 = standard deviation of the *Phantom* method for the sitting height (cm).
- 109.35 = sum of the mode of Antero-posterior chest depth + Transverse chest breadth + Corrected waist girth of the *Phantom* method (cm).
- 7.09 = sum of the standard deviations for Antero-posterior chest depth + Transverse chest breadth + Corrected waist girth of the *Phantom* method (cm).

$$\begin{aligned}3\text{rd Residual mass(kg)} = {} & (\text{Z Residual} * 1.24) \\ & + 6.1/(89.92/\text{Sitting height (cm)})^3\end{aligned}$$

where:
- 1.24 = standard deviation of the *Phantom* method for the residual mass (kg).
- 6.1 = mode of the *Phantom* method for the residual mass (kg).
- 89.92 = mode of the *Phantom* method for the sitting height (cm).

In the event that it is not possible to address body composition by this method, either due to measurement time or the anthropometrist's training in terms of variables that they know how to measure, the alternative could be a four-compartment model without mixing models. Thus, the following equations would be performed:

- Adipose component: Kerr (1991). The measurement of the triceps, subscapular, supraspinal, abdominal, thigh and calf skinfolds is necessary.

$$1\text{st } \Sigma \text{ 6 skinfolds} = \text{Triceps skinfold (mm)} + \text{Subscapular skinfold (mm)}$$

$$+ \text{Supraspinal skinfold (mm)} + \text{Abdominal skinfold (mm)} + \text{Thigh skinfold (mm)} + \text{Calf skinfold (mm)}$$

$$\text{2nd Z adiposity} = [\Sigma\ 6\ \text{skinfolds} * (170.18/\text{Stretch stature (cm)}) - 116.41]/34.79$$

where:
- 170.18 = mode of the *Phantom* method for stretch stature (cm).
- 116.41 = sum of the mode of the skinfolds of the *Phantom* method (mm).
- 34.79 = sum of the standard deviations for the skinfolds of the *Phantom* method (mm).

$$\text{3rd Adipose mass (kg)} = \left[(\text{Z adiposity} * 5.85) + 25.6\right]/(170.18/\text{Stretch stature (cm)})^3$$

where:
- 5.85 = standard deviation of the *Phantom* method for the adipose mass (kg).
- 25.6 = mode of the *Phantom* method for the adipose mass (kg).
- 170.18 = mode of the *Phantom* method for stretch stature (cm).

- Skeletal muscle mass: Lee's formula (2000). The measurement of stretch stature, arm relaxed, thigh middle and calf girths, and the triceps, thigh and calf skinfolds are required.

$$\begin{aligned}\text{Skeletal muscle mass (kg)} = {} & \text{Stretch stature (m)} * (0.00744 \\ & * \text{Corrected arm girth (cm)}^2 \\ & + 0.00088 * \text{Corrected thigh girth (cm)}^2 \\ & + 0.00441 * \text{Corrected calf girth (cm)}^2 \\ & + (2.4 * \text{sex}) - 0.048 * \text{age (years)} \\ & + \text{ethnicity} + 7.8\end{aligned}$$

where:
- Corrected arm girth = Arm relaxed girth (cm) – (π * (triceps skinfold (cm)).
- Corrected thigh girth = Thigh middle girth (cm) – (π * (thigh skinfold (cm)).
- Corrected calf girth = Calf girth (cm) – (π * (calf skinfold (cm)).
- Sex = 1 men; 0 women.
- Ethnicity = – 2 Asians and; 1.1 African-Americans; 0 Caucasians and Hispanics.

- Bone mass: Rocha's formula (1975) should be used for any population, except for the elderly. The measurement of stretch stature, the bi-styloid breadth and the femur breadth are required.

$$\text{Bone mass (kg)} = 3.02 * (\text{Stretch stature (m)}^2 * \text{Bi} - \text{styloid breadth (m)} * \text{Femur breadth (m)} * 400)^{0.712}$$

Regarding the elderly population, it is advised to use the equation by Martin (1991). For this, it is necessary to measure the stretch stature, the humerus, bi-styloid, femur and bi-malleolar breadths.

$$\text{Bone mass (kg)} = 0.00006 * \text{Stretch stature (cm)} * (\text{Humerus breadth (cm)} + \text{Bi} - \text{styloid breadth (cm)} + \text{Femur breadth (cm)} + \text{Bimalleolar breadth (cm)})^2$$

- Residual mass: remaining amount, assuming that error will be introduced, but it is less because components are not mixed.

The third alternative would be to address body composition through a two-compartment model, where lipid mass is estimated with a suitable formula for the population evaluated, that is, with a formula that has been validated in a population similar to the one intended to be evaluated, then indicating that the rest of the mass is lipid-free mass. This approach may be interesting when the focus of the assessment is exclusively adiposity.

5.6 Sum of Skinfolds

As has been observed so far, the estimation of body composition using the different methods and existing formulas presents many limitations. Despite this, through anthropometry, body composition can be estimated in a valid and reliable way, with a good balance between assessment time and data provided, as long as the considerations and limitations of this method are considered.

However, in recent years, there has been a new trend in the estimation of body composition with anthropometry, promoted in both the scientific field and in field work, which proposes complementing the analysis of body composition with the data of the sum of at least 5 skinfolds from different parts of the body, expressed in their original units (mm) as a variable of adiposity.

This sum of skinfolds can be accompanied by a profile of skinfolds (graphical representation of each of the skinfolds in a line graph), which allows knowing exactly the place where a subject is modifying his/her adiposity. This aspect is interesting in the sports field, but also in the field of health because the accumulation of fat in certain areas of the body is strongly related to the onset of chronic diseases.

In conclusion, the sum of skinfolds could be a good alternative as a representative of adiposity, without the disadvantages of estimating adipose tissue/fat mass/lipid mass being present.

5.7 Corrected Girths

As with the estimation of adiposity with body composition methods, there are limitations in the estimation of the muscular component. As a result, the use corrected girths as a complementary variable in the assessment of the muscular component has recently been proposed. The corrected girths are so named because what is done is to subtract the subcutaneous fat from the measured girth, with this being the value of the skinfold. This allows for the corrected girth to correspond to the muscle and bone development in the arm, thigh and calf, although with a small margin of error belonging to the vascular and lymphatic system. Since bones have very little growth in the transverse direction in a short space of time, it can be assumed that changes in the corrected girths are due to a change in the muscle development of the area. Not in vain, the estimation of muscle mass in anthropometry is based on the calculation of corrected girths in its formulas.

Thus, the following corrected girths can be calculated:

- Corrected arm girth: arm relaxed girth (cm) − π * triceps skinfold (cm).
- Corrected thigh girth: thigh middle girth (cm) − π * thigh skinfold (cm).
- Corrected calf girth: calf girth (cm) − π * calf skinfold (cm).

The corrected girths of the limbs (corrected arm, thigh middle and calf) include two from the trunk, corrected chest girth, and corrected waist girth.

The formulas are as follows:

- Corrected chest girth: chest girth (cm) − π * subscapular skinfold (cm).
- Corrected waist girth: waist girth (cm) − π * abdominal skinfold (cm).

Both trunk girths are more related to health than to sports performance, as they do not deal strongly with muscle development, but refer to the organs and the accumulation of visceral fat. Thus, the corrected chest girth deals with the accumulation of fat near the heart, while the waist corrected indicates the accumulation of fat near the digestive organs. However, it should be noted that we are correcting both girths with skinfolds that do not go in the same direction as the measured girth. In addition, the waist girth, following the ISAK methodology, is not taken in the same place as the abdominal skinfold, except in overweight and obese people in whom the minimum waist size cannot be found. In these cases, it is taken in the middle area between the iliac crest and the lateral lower rib edge (10th rib), which does coincide with the abdominal skinfold. Therefore, this girth is very useful in people with overweightness and obesity, as a decrease in the corrected girth of the waist will indicate a decrease in visceral fat in this area.

With the corrected girths, the cross-sectional muscle areas (CMA) can be calculated:

$$\text{Cross-sectional muscle area (CMA)} = \text{Corrected girth} * \text{Corrected girth}/(4 * \pi)$$

The use of corrected girths is not without limitations. In the calculation of the corrected girths, a series of issues are assumed such as the girths being completely round, the skinfolds presenting the same density and distribution around the girth, or that the skin having a constant thickness, with these issues not being entirely correct. However, these issues are constant in all subjects and, therefore, the same error is always made. Thus, these limitations can be assumed and the corrected girths can be used as an alternative to the knowledge of the development musculoskeletal in a segmental manner.

5.8 Conclusions on the Estimation of Body Composition

In conclusion, the methods available for the assessment of the body composition are numerous and, although not interchangeable, seem valid if their limitations and considerations are taken into account. Regarding the anthropometric method, the sum of skinfolds and the corrected girths seem to be the best option to assess the body composition of subjects as a complement to the estimation of body composition, by solving a large part of the problems observed in the application of formulas.

5.9 Questionnaire

1. Using the anthropometric method, it is possible to calculate body composition variables:
   (a) It is true, as long as the protocol is strictly followed.
   (b) They can be estimated, but not calculated because it is not a direct method.
   (c) They can be calculated only with certain formulas.
   (d) It is not possible in any way to calculate the components of body composition.
2. Within the models of body composition estimation, the tissue model:
   (a) Divides the body based on the chemical elements that compose it.
   (b) Divides the body into molecules based on the micro and macronutrients that compose it.
   (c) It is a model of body composition that allows the addressing body composition through tissues.
   (d) Breaks down the body according to the cells that compose it.

3. A common error in terminology when discussing body composition from the tissue model is to use:
   (a) Fat mass instead of adipose tissue.
   (b) Muscle tissue instead of protein mass.
   (c) Bone mass instead of residual mass.
   (d) None of the above is true.
4. Among the most used methods to assess body composition:
   (a) Cadaver dissection is the only direct method.
   (b) Cadaver dissection has served as a validation method for subsequent indirect methods.
   (c) Various experts in anthropometry have based their research on the results of William Ross's dissection studies.
   (d) All are true.
5. Within the indirect methods of estimating body composition, indicate the false one:
   (a) DXA is the reference method for estimating adiposity.
   (b) Hydrostatic weighing studies body composition from the molecular model, calculating the body density of the individual.
   (c) Plethysmography estimates lipid mass and lipid-free mass.
   (d) Bioelectrical impedance bases its estimates on the conductivity of the different components of the body.
6. Anthropometry as a method of estimating body composition:
   (a) It is a less reliable method than other indirect methods.
   (b) Can address body composition from the atomic model.
   (c) There are various equations for estimating body composition that can be used with anthropometric variables.
   (d) Anthropometry cannot be used in the estimation of body composition.
7. From the anthropometric method, body composition can be approached from a model:
   (a) Two-compartment (two components).
   (b) Four-compartment (four components).
   (c) Five-compartment (five components).
   (d) All are true.
8. Taking into account the characteristics of indirect methods of estimating body composition, it should be noted that:
   (a) The data obtained through different estimation methods can be compared.
   (b) Different estimation equations can be used and the data compared, as long as the method is the same.
   (c) Some of the anthropometric formulas have been validated in a certain population, which limits that they can only be used in a population with similar characteristics.
   (d) Bioimpedance is a method considered very reliable for analysing individuals.

9. Due to the advantages and disadvantages of the anthropometric method, when intending to address the analysis of body composition, it is recommended to use the model:
   (a) Five-compartment.
   (b) Six-compartment.
   (c) Two-compartment.
   (d) Four-compartment.
10. Due to the different errors that can arise regarding the analysis of body composition from the anthropometric method:
   (a) It is recommended to mix components obtained with different methods when estimating body composition.
   (b) The estimation formulas do not introduce any type of error in the calculation of body composition.
   (c) It is recommended to use the sum of skinfolds and corrected girths in the assessment of body composition due to their reduced error compared to formulas.
   (d) None of the above is true.

Answers:
1.b 2.c 3.a 4.d 5.a 6.c 7.d 8.c 9.a 10.c

Bibliography

Boughman, J. K., Masters, M. A., Morgan, C. A., Ruden, T. M., & Rochelle, S. G. (2019). Assessing the validity of bioelectrical impedance and skinfold calipers for measuring body composition in NOLS backcountry hikers. *Wilderness & Environmental Medicine, 30*(4), 369–377.

Carter, J. (1982). Body composition of Montreal Olympic athletes. In J. Carter (Ed.), *Physical structure of Olympic athletes part I: The Montreal Olympic games anthropological project*. Karger.

Doran, D. A., Mc Geever, S., Collins, K. D., Quinn, C., McElhone, R., & Scott, M. (2014). The validity of commonly used adipose tissue body composition equations relative to dual energy X-ray absorptiometry (DXA) in gaelic games players. *International Journal of Sports Medicine, 35*(2), 95–100.

Durnin, J. V., & Womersley, J. (1974). Body fat assessed from total body density and its estimation from skinfold thickness: Measurements on 481 men and women aged from 16 to 72 years. *British Journal of Nutrition, 32*(1), 77–97.

Faulkner, J. (1968). Physiology of swimming and diving. In H. Falls (Ed.), *Exercise physiology*. Academic Press.

Jackson, A. S., & Pollock, M. L. (1978). Generalised equations for predicting body density of men. *British Journal of Nutrition, 40*, 497–504.

Kasper, A. M., Langan-Evans, C., Hudson, J. F., Brownlee, T. E., Harper, L. D., Naughton, R. J., Morton, J. P., & Close, G. L. (2021). Come back skinfolds, all is forgiven: A narrative review of the efficacy of common body composition methods in applied sports practice. *Nutrients, 13*(4), 1075.

Leal, L., Barbosa, G., Ferreira, R., Avelino, E. B., Bezerra, A. N., Vale, S., & Maciel, B. (2019). Cross-validation of prediction equations for estimating body composition in ballet dancers. *PLoS ONE, 14*(7), e0219045.

Martin, A. (1991). Anthropometric assessment of bone mineral. In J. Himes (Ed.), *Anthropometric assessment of nutritional status* (pp. 185–196). Wiley-Liss.

Mecherques-Carini, M., Esparza-Ros, F., Albaladejo-Saura, M., & Vaquero-Cristóbal, R. (2022). Agreement and differences between fat estimation formulas using kinanthropometry in a physically active population. *Applied Sciences, 12*(24), 13043.

Nickerson, B. S., Snarr, R. L., & Ryan, G. A. (2019). Validity of foot-to-foot bioelectrical impedance for estimating body composition in NCAA Division I male athletes: A 3-compartment model comparison. *Journal of Strength and Conditioning Research, 33*(12), 3361–3366.

Nickerson, B. S., McLester, C. N., McLester, J. R., & Kliszczewicz, B. M. (2020). Agreement between 2 segmental bioimpedance devices, BOD POD, and DXA in obese adults. *Journal of Clinical Densitometry, 23*(1), 138–148.

Reiter, R., Iglseder, B., Treschnitzer, W., Alzner, R., Mayr-Pirker, B., Kreutzer, M., Pirich, C., Kässmann, H., Dovjak, P., & Reiss, J. (2019). Quantifying appendicular muscle mass in geriatric inpatients: Performance of different single frequency BIA equations in comparison to dual X-ray absorptiometry. *Archives of Gerontology and Geriatrics, 80*, 98–103.

Ross, W. D., & Kerr, D. A. (1991). Fractionation of body mass: a new method for use in clinical nutrition and sports medicine. *Apunts. Medicina de l´Esport, 18*(1), 175–187.

Schubert, M. M., Seay, R. F., Spain, K. K., Clarke, H. E., & Taylor, J. K. (2019). Reliability and validity of various laboratory methods of body composition assessment in young adults. *Clinical Physiology and Functional Imaging, 39*(2), 150–159.

Vaquero-Cristóbal, R., Albaladejo-Saura, M., Luna-Badachi, A. E., & Esparza-Ros, F. (2020). Differences in fat mass estimation formulas in physically active adult population and relationship with sums of skinfolds. *International Journal of Environmental Research and Public Health, 17*(21), 7777.

Withers, R., Craig, N., Bourdon, P., & Norton, K. (1987). Relative body fat and anthropometric prediction of body density of male athletes. *European Journal of Applied Physiology and Occupational Physiology, 56*(2), 191–200.

Analysis of Proportionality Through Anthropometric Assessment

6

Abstract

Proportionality is the branch of knowledge that analyses the relationship between different parts of the body or between the body and some reference to determine their relative size. There are two main types of proportionality: body indices and comparison with a reference model. Within the body indices, we find: (a) relative measurements or proportions, such as the relative sitting height, relative arm span, relative upper limb length, relative lower limb length, and waist-to-height index; (b) indices such as the intermembral index, brachial index, acromial-iliac index, crural index, thoracic index, waist-hip index and fat distribution index; (c) ponderal indices or robustness indices, highlighting the Quetelet index or body mass index, Bouchard index, and ponderal index. This chapter explains what each one consists of, the formula to calculate them, and how to interpret their results. Next, the comparison with the reference model, also known as Phantom model, is presented. This model was created to compare an individual's anthropometric variables with those of a reference population. It specifies how to calculate the Phantom model value step by step, as well as how to interpret it.

Keywords

Body indices • Relative measurements • Indices • Ponderal indices • Robustness indices • Phantom • Waist-hip ratio • Waist-to-height ratio • Body mass index

6.1 Definition

Proportionality was defined by Carter as the branch of knowledge responsible for analysing the relationship between the various body parts, or the relationship of the whole body with respect to some reference to find its relative size.

© The Author(s), under exclusive license to Springer Nature Switzerland AG 2025

F. Esparza-Ros and R. Vaquero-Cristóbal, *Anthropometry*,
https://doi.org/10.1007/978-3-031-77535-2_6

6.2 Fields of Application of Proportionality

Proportionality is applicable to different fields of knowledge, with the first of the fields where it was developed being the field of sports performance. Indeed, when analysing elite subjects of the same sport, it can be observed that proportionally, they all share certain characteristics, such as whether their arms and legs are short, average, or long, as compared to stretch stature; the shape of their trunk when comparing its width at shoulder level or at hip level; or if they have high, average, or low body mass with respect to their stretch stature, among others.

But sports performance is not the only area of application of proportionality. Another of the branches where this topic has been most developed is ergonomics. Ergonomics is defined as the scientific discipline of designing workstations, processes, and products that humans can use efficiently, easily and safely, optimising health and comfort. It is based on anatomical, physiological, and psychological aspects. More specifically, when ergonomically designing furniture, infrastructure, clothing, means of transport, etc., the anthropometric characteristics of the target population are taken into account so that they can be used efficiently and maintain adequate postural hygiene. Thus, for example, anthropometric proportionality variables are taken into account when designing the height of the seats of chairs, so that they are at a height at which the majority of the population can sit with their legs bent at 90° and their feet are supported; or in the case of doors, they are designed so that people can pass comfortably both in terms of width and height but at the same time without being too large so that they are energy efficient, limiting the loss of heat or cold.

6.3 Proportionality Models

Among the most commonly used proportionality variables, we find two main blocks. The first block is characterised by the variables being related within the same subject, and are called body indices. With this block of variables, it will be possible to know if the subject has a proportionally larger or smaller variable than another, with the variables being compared with those from the individual themselves.

The second major block is the comparison with a reference model. This allows for the comparison of anthropometric variables with the population, to find if the subject has a large, average, or small variable as compared to the rest of the subjects.

Next, the two blocks of proportionality variables will be described.

Table 6.1 Classification of the relative sitting height for men and women

Relative sitting height	Reference values for men (%)	Reference values for women (%)
Short trunk	< 50.9	< 51.9
Medium trunk	51 a 52.9	52 a 53.9
Long trunk	≥ 53	≥ 54

6.3.1 Body Indices

A body index is defined as the relationship between two body measurements expressed as a percentage of the smaller over the larger. They are useful for verifying if a certain variable is relative or proportionally large or small as compared to another in a certain percentage. Among the different indices, three types can be distinguished: relative measurements, indices, and ponderal indices or robustness. Each of these blocks will be discussed below.

6.3.1.1 Relative Measurement

These are proportionality variables in which a certain measurement is relativised (numerator) with respect to stretch stature (denominator) in the form of a percentage of the first with respect to the second. Among them we find.

Relative Sitting Height

The relative sitting height is the relationship of the length of the head plus the trunk with respect to stretch stature. It allows to relativise the size of the body from the hip upwards and from the hip downwards. In this way, it will be possible to observe if a subject has a proportionally short trunk, and therefore a long lower limb; a proportional trunk and lower limb; or a long trunk and, therefore, a proportionally short lower limb. To calculate the relative sitting height, the following equation is used:

$$\text{Relative sitting height} = (\text{Sitting Height (cm)}/\text{Stretch stature (cm)}) * 100$$

Regarding the relative sitting height, men and women are not proportionally the same. Generally, men have proportionally longer lower limbs than women, and for this reason, a differentiation is applied to the reference values of this index with respect to sex. The classification of the relative sitting height can be found in Table 6.1.

Regarding the relationship of the relative sitting height with sports performance, a proportionally short trunk, accompanied therefore by a proportionally long lower limb, will benefit modalities where running predominates; while a proportionally long trunk and, therefore, a proportionally short lower limb, will benefit the modalities in which having the centre of gravity close to the ground for greater stability is a competitive advantage.

Relative Arm Span

The relative arm span refers to the relationship between the arm span and stretch stature. It allows relativising how wide a subject can be with their arms open at 90° with how tall they are. The mathematical expression for its calculation is as follows:

$$\text{Relative Arm Span} = (\text{Arm Span (cm)}/\text{Stretch stature (cm)}) * 100$$

Women commonly have an arm span that is slightly less than their stretch stature, which results in reported relative arm span of < 100%. In contrast, men usually have a 1:1 ratio, meaning that arm span and stretch stature are often similar, which reports values in the relative arm span of around 100%.

However, one thing to bear in mind is that arm span is modifiable, as it not only depends on bone variables, but is also influenced by the ability of the muscles, the muscle–tendon system, and the ligament system, to perform a scapular abduction. Therefore, this variable that can be modified to some extent with training. Thus, in sports where scapular abduction is a common gesture, such as all sports that involve throwing or hitting implements with the upper limb, such as basketball, handball, volleyball, water polo, athletics throws, etc.; or where propulsion is performed with the upper limbs, such as swimming, you can find subjects with much larger arm spans than their stretch stature. This high relative arm span also provides a competitive advantage in these types of modalities.

On the other hand, subjects who have Marfan syndrome usually have arm spans also much larger than their stretch stature, but this syndrome cannot be diagnosed based solely on arm span, so genetic tests must be used for its diagnosis.

Relative Length of the Upper Limb

The relative length of the upper limb is a variable that allows us to discover if the upper limb is short, medium or long in relation to stretch stature. To calculate it, it is first necessary to know the length of the upper limb. This is done through the upper arm (acromiale-radiale length), forearm (radiale-stylion length), and hand (midstylion-dactylion length) segments. By dividing the sum of these three segments by the stretch stature, you can verify the relative length of the upper limb. The mathematical expression of the calculation is as follows:

$$\begin{aligned}\text{Relative length of the upper limb} = {} & [(\text{Acromiale} - \text{radiale length (cm)} \\ & + \text{Radiale} - \text{stylion length (cm)} \\ & + \text{Midstylion} - \text{dactylion length (cm)}) \\ & /\text{Stretch stature (cm)}] * 100\end{aligned}$$

Table 6.2 presents the values with which to classify the relative length of the upper limb.

Regarding the relationship of the relative length of the upper limb with sports performance, a long upper limb is a competitive advantage in sports such as swimming, throwing sports, or in team sports such as basketball, volleyball, or handball.

Table 6.2 Classification of the relative length of the upper limb

Relative length of the upper limb	Reference values (%)
Short upper limbs	< 44.9
Medium upper limbs	45 a 46.9
Long upper limbs	≥ 47

Table 6.3 Classification of the relative length of the lower limb

Relative length of the lower limb	Reference values (%)
Short lower limbs	< 54.9
Medium lower limbs	55 a 56.9
Long lower limbs	≥ 57

On the other hand, a proportionally short upper limb gives a competitive advantage in weightlifting, in which it is an advantage that the distance of the load to the centre of the axis, which is the trunk, is as small as possible.

Relative Length of the Lower Limb

The relative length of the lower limb is a variable that allows us to discover if the lower limb is short, medium or long in relation to stretch stature. For this, it is first necessary to know the length of the lower limb. For the measurement of the length of the lower limb, the iliospinale height will be used, as it is the approximate height at which the head of the femur is located. The tronchanterion height will not be taken, as the greater trochanter is not located at the top of the femur, but below its head. The mathematical expression for the calculation of the relative length of the lower limb is as follows:

$$\text{Relative length of the lower limb} = [\text{Iliospinale height (cm)} / \text{Stretch stature (cm)}] * 100$$

Table 6.3 contains the values with which to classify the relative length of the lower limb.

Regarding the relationship of the relative length of the lower limb with sports performance, a proportionally large lower limb length will benefit modalities where running predominates, while a proportionally short length will benefit modalities in which it is a competitive advantage to have the centre of gravity close to the ground for greater stability.

Waist-to-Height Index

The waist-to-height index relates the waist girth with the individual's stretch stature. An important issue to consider in relation to this index is the place that is taken as reference for the waist measurement. Thus, while some organisations such as the International Society for the Advancement of Kinanthropometry (ISAK) advocate for the measurement of this girth at the smallest part of the waist, other manuals and societies have proposed the assessment of this girth at the midpoint

Table 6.4 Classification of the waist-to-height ratio according to age

Waist-to-height ratio	Reference values for the under 40s (%)	Reference values between 40 and 50 years (%)	Reference values for the over 50s (%)
Normality	≤ 50	≤ 55	≤ 60
Cardiovascular risk	> 50	> 55	> 60

Table 6.5 Classification of the waist-to-height ratio in growing boys and girls

Waist-to-height ratio	Reference values for boys	Reference values for girls
Severe thinness	≤ 0.34	≤ 0.34
Slight thinness	0.35 to 0.42	0.35 to 0.41
Normal weight	0.43 to 0.52	0.42 to 0.48
Overweight	0.53 to 0.57	0.49 to 0.53
Obesity	0.58 to 0.62	0.54 to 0.57
Morbid obesity	≥ 0.63	≥ 0.58

between the lowermost part of the last rib and the upper edge of the iliac crest, or by the measurement at the height of the omphalion (navel), among others. This aspect could modify the values found, so it has to be taken into consideration when talking about reference values and classifying this index.

This index has traditionally been used as a measurement of the distribution of body fat and, therefore, is related to the risk of obesity and suffering from cardiovascular diseases, among others. The mathematical expression for the calculation of the waist-to-height index is as follows:

$$\text{Waist-to-height index} = [\text{Waist girth (cm)}/\text{Stretch stature (cm)}] * 100$$

Table 6.4 shows the values with which to classify the waist-to-height index based on age.

In addition, it has also been used in the growing population, as it allows comparing individuals with different stretch statures. Table 6.5 shows the reference values to consider for its application in infants and adolescents.

6.3.1.2 Index

An index is a relationship between two anthropometric variables among which stretch stature is not found.

Intermembral Index

This index provides information regarding the proportionality of the length of the upper limb in relation to the length of the lower limb. For the calculation of the length of the upper limb, the length of the upper arm (acromiale-radiale length), forearm (radiale-stylion length) and hand (midstylion-dactylion length) should be

Table 6.6 Classification of the brachial index

Brachial index	Reference values (%)
Short forearm	< 78
Medium forearm	78 a 82.9
Long forearm	≥ 83

added. On the other hand, for the measurement of the lower limb, the iliospinale height will be used. The formula for its calculation is:

$$\text{Intermembral index} = (\text{Upper limb length (cm)} / \text{Lower limb length (cm)}) * 100$$

Regarding values, in the case of women, the upper limb usually represents around 80% of the lower limb, while in men, it is normal for the upper limb to represent 82.5% of the lower limb.

Regarding the relationship of the intermembral index with sports performance, that the length of the upper limb is proportionally longer than the length of the lower limb will be an advantage in those sports in which propulsion depends on the upper limb, as in the case of swimming; while a lower limb proportionally longer than the upper limb will be a competitive advantage in running and jumping sports where there are no throws, hits, etc. with the upper limb, as may be the case of running modalities in athletics.

Brachial Index

This index refers to the relationship between the length of the arm (acromiale-radiale length) and the forearm (radiale-stylion length). This index provides information as to whether the forearm is long, average, or short, in relation to the arm. Its mathematical expression is the following:

$$\text{Brachial index} = (\text{Radiale-stylion length (cm)} / \text{Acromiale-radiale length (cm)}) * 100$$

Normal values for the brachial index can be found in Table 6.6.

Regarding the relationship of the brachial index with sports performance, a large brachial index, that is, a proportionally large forearm in relation to the arm, will benefit sports where the axis of movement is the elbow. This is because, by moving away from the lever arm, it provides more axis length, and applying the same force generates a greater torque, as can be the case of a baseball swing or the grip phase when swimming in freestyle. On the contrary, a low brachial index, that is, the forearm is proportionally short in relation to the arm, will benefit sports where the movement starts from the shoulder, such as in a tennis serve, or in weightlifting, where it is better for the athlete to move the load the minimum distance possible away from the shoulder.

Table 6.7 Classification of the acromial-iliac index

Acromial-iliac index	Reference values for pre-pubertals (%)	Reference values for post-pubertal men (%)	Reference values for post-pubertal women (%)
Trapezoidal trunk	< 69.9	< 69.9	< 79.9
Intermediate trunk	70 to 74.9	70 to 74.9	80 to 84.9
Rectangular trunk	≥ 75	≥ 75	≥ 85

Acromial-Iliac Index

This index refers to the relationship between the biiliocristal breadth and the biacromial breadth. It provides information on the difference between the width of the shoulders (biacromial breadth) and the hips (biiliocristal breadth), which allows us to know the shape of the trunk. Its mathematical expression is the following:

$$\text{Acromial-iliac index} = (\text{Biiliocristal breadth (cm)} / \text{Biacromial breadth (cm)}) * 100$$

The biiliocristal breadth is placed in the numerator since, in most cases, people have a larger biacromial breadth than biiliocristal.

Depending on the proportionality between both breadths, different body shapes can be distinguished. The classification of the acromial-iliac index is found in Table 6.7. It should be noted that once puberty is passed, a sexual dimorphism occurs in the width of the hips, increasing to a greater extent in women than in men. This is because, in the case of women, during puberty, the bone structures that make up the pelvis adapt for a potential childbirth, consequently increasing the biiliocristal breadth. Therefore, the classification varies between men and women starting from this moment.

Regarding the relationship of the acromial-iliac index and sports performance, a trapezoidal trunk, characterized by a greater width of shoulders than hips, will benefit in sports such as swimming; while a rectangular trunk, characterized by a greater width of hips compared to the shoulders, will benefit in those sports in which being stable is a competitive advantage and, therefore, it is better for the mass to be more localized to the hip area, because it is closer to the centre of gravity, such as in sumo wrestling or weightlifting.

Crural Index

The crural index refers to the relationship between the length of the leg and the thigh. However, there is some controversy regarding the measurement to take as a reference for the length of the thigh and the leg. The most commonly used method for its calculation uses the length of the leg, the tibiale mediale-sphyrion tibiale length, while for the length of the thigh the reference is the trochanterion-tibiale laterale length. However, the reality is that the length of the trochanterion-tibiale laterale, does not fully correspond with the length of the thigh, as the measurement begins at the greater trochanter, not taking into account the head of the femur. For this reason, some authors propose taking the iliospinale height and subtracting the tibiale-laterale height to obtain the real length of the thigh. In any case, what is really important when measuring this variable, is to do it in the same way as it was done in the reference with which you want to make a comparison. In the case that such a reference does not exist, it could be faster to measure the length of the thigh as the length of the trochanterion-tibiale laterale, knowing the limitation of this measurement, as previously indicated. The formula for the calculation of the crural index is:

$$\text{Crural index} = (\text{Leg length (cm)}/\text{Thigh length (cm)}) * 100$$

Due to the different formulas that exist to estimate the length of the thigh in the application of this index, no values are proposed, since the value of the index will depend on the length that is used in representation of the length of the thigh. On the other hand, if you want to compare this value with that of a reference, the length of the thigh must be measured in the same way so that the comparison can be made.

Regarding the relationship of the crural index with sports performance, a large crural index, that is, a proportionally long leg with respect to the thigh will benefit sports in which the axis of movement is the knee. This is because, by moving away from the lever arm, it provides more axis length so that with the same power, more force is achieved. This could be the case of a ball kick in football. On the contrary, a low crural index, that is, the leg is proportionally short with respect to the thigh, will benefit sports in which the movement starts from the hip, such as the propulsion of the legs when swimming freestyle or backstroke.

Thoracic Index

The thoracic index refers to the proportionality of the antero-posterior chest dept and transverse chest breadth. It is an index related to the proportions of the rib cage. Its mathematical expression is as follows:

$$\text{Thoracic index} = (\text{Antero-posterior chest depth (cm)} \\ /\text{Transverse chest breadth (cm)}) * 100$$

It has been observed that the value of the thoracic index varies unevenly throughout adolescence depending on sex, as it is strongly associated to the size of the lungs and their expansion during breathing. Thus, while in the case of girls it remains relatively stable throughout adolescence, even slightly decreasing at some point; in the case of boys it increases gradually with age.

Regarding the relationship of the thoracic index with sports performance, it must be taken into consideration that this index increases with sports training, especially with aerobic training. As a result of the above, this index is commonly higher in aerobic sports. In this type of sports, cardiopulmonary adaptations occur, and this increase also occurs structurally at the cardiac and pulmonary level.

Table 6.8 Classification of the waist-hip ratio as a function of sex

Waist-hip ratio	Reference values for men	Reference values for women
Normality	< 1.00	< 0.80
Abdominal obesity	≥ 1.00	≥ 0.80

Waist-Hip Ratio

This index refers to the relationship between the waist and hips girths. It is an index widely used in the field of health for its important correlation with the onset of non-communicable diseases such as obesity and cardiovascular diseases, as it is an indicative index of abdominal fat accumulation. However, an important issue to consider regarding this index is the place that is taken as a reference for the measurement of both girths. Thus, there is a great debate in the protocol to follow for the measurement of the waist girth, and while some organisations such as the International Society for the Advancement of the Kinanthropometry (ISAK) advocates for the measurement of this girth at the smallest part of the waist, other manuals and societies have proposed the assessment of this girth at the midpoint between the lowest part of the last rib and the upper edge of the iliac crest, or by measuring at the height of the omphalion (navel), among other variants. Not in vain, ISAK advocates for measuring the girth at the midpoint between the last rib and the upper edge of the iliac crest in those cases where the smallest part of the waist cannot be observed. Regarding the measurement of the hips girth, the greatest debate seems to focus on the position of the legs (together or apart) to measure it, which could significantly influence the result. These aspects could modify the values found in the measurement of both girths, so they should be taken into consideration when discussing the values and classifying this index.

Its calculation is obtained from the division of the waist girth by the hips girth. Its mathematical expression is as follows:

$$\text{Waist-hip ratio} = \text{Waist girth (cm)}/\text{hips girth (cm)}$$

In Table 6.8, the normal values of the waist-hip index are found according to sex.

Fat Distribution Index

The fat distribution index refers to the relationship between the adipose tissue accumulated in the limbs and the adipose tissue accumulated in the trunk, measured through triceps, thigh, and leg skinfolds, in the case of the limbs; and subscapular, supraspinal and abdominal skinfolds in the case of the trunk. Its mathematical expression is as follows:

$$\begin{aligned}\text{Fat distribution index} = {} & (\text{Triceps skinfold (mm)} + \text{Thigh skinfold (mm)} \\ & + \text{Leg skinfold (mm)})/(\text{Subscapular skinfold (mm)} \\ & + \text{Supraspinal skinfold (mm)} + \text{Abdominal skinfold (mm)})\end{aligned}$$

It is important to consider that men tend to accumulate more fat in the trunk area than in the limbs, while women tend to accumulate more in the limbs.

Regarding the relationship of the fat distribution index with sports performance, a distribution of fat centred in the trunk can be a competitive advantage in men sports as compared to women, because the accumulation of fat in the trunk provides greater stability in most sports and greater efficiency in mobilising the limbs, which occurs in all sports. This does not mean that a greater amount of fat is beneficial, but within the fat possessed by this type of athlete, it is a competitive advantage that this fat be in the trunk.

6.3.1.3 Ponderal Indices or Robustness Indices

The ponderal indices relate body mass to stretch stature, regardless of the mathematical operation performed with these two variables. Therefore, these indices show the proportional relationship between body mass and stretch stature.

Before addressing the body mass indices, it is necessary to consider the limitations of using body mass in these indices. The fact is that the body mass variable does not differentiate between muscle content and fat content. In addition, if the focus of most of these indices is health, we find that in these indices, an excess of body mass in relation to stretch stature is interpreted as an excess of adiposity, when it might not be so. This should be taken into account when applied to populations where muscle mass predominates, such as athletes.

Among the ponderal indices or robustness indices, you can find.

Quetelet Index or Body Mass Index (BMI)

This index was created by Adolphe Quetelet in 1832, a Belgian mathematician and statistician interested in statistical studies, using data from European men, although this index is globally known as the body mass index. To calculate the body mass index, the body mass is divided by the individual's stretch stature squared. Its mathematical expression is as follows:

$$\text{BMI} = \text{Body mass (kg)}/\text{Stretch stature (m)}^2$$

This index has widespread acceptance worldwide, to the point of being used by international organisations to classify individuals based on their body mass. The most commonly used classification is promoted by the World Health Organisation, which categorises subjects based on the values shown in Table 6.9.

However, despite it being a widely used index due to its simplicity and easy application, this index is not without limitations. One of them is that, in this index, the body mass, which occupies three dimensions, as it has width, length and depth, is divided by the stretch stature, which is a one-dimensional variable. By squaring it, a second dimension is applied to the stretch stature, and the problem arises when relating a three-dimensional variable with a two-dimensional one. As a result, the changes that occur in both variables do not maintain proportionality, so it is less sensitive to changes in body mass than in stretch stature.

Table 6.9 Classification of the body mass index (BMI)

Body mass index	Reference values
Underweight	< 18.5
Normal weight	18.5–24.9
Overweight	25.0–29.9
Obesity type 1	30.0–34.9
Obesity type 2	35.0–39.9
Obesity type 3	> 40.0

Bouchard Index

The Bouchard index relates body mass to stretch stature without applying any correction to the variables. Its mathematical expression is:

$$\text{Bouchard Index} = \text{Body mass (kg)}/\text{Stretch stature (cm)}$$

In this case, the body mass is divided by the individual's stretch stature, so it relates a three-dimensional variable with a one-dimensional one. This makes the sensitivity to changes even lower, so this index does not provide a better proportionality relationship than the BMI, and is therefore hardly used.

Ponderal Index

This index multiplies the body mass in grams by 100, to then divide it by the stretch stature (cm) cubed. Its mathematical expression is:

$$\text{Ponderal Index} = (\text{body mass (g)} * 100)/\text{stretch stature (cm)}^3$$

This is the robustness index that best maintains dimensionality. The body mass has three dimensions, and the stretch stature is cubed, which results in three dimensions as well. In this way, this index will detect changes proportionally in body mass or stretch stature, which the other robustness indices would not be able to detect. On the contrary, the numerical results of this index are much less intuitive than those of the BMI, as they are very small numbers, and therefore more difficult to interpret.

6.3.2 Comparison with a Reference Model

For the comparison of an individual's variables with those of the population in order to find if their variable is proportionally larger, equal, or smaller, the *Phantom* model is used. The *Phantom* model was created in 1974 as a proposal to address the existing problem in anthropometry regarding the need for a comparative reference model.

The *Phantom* model was created with data from large population anthropometric studies. Data from studies in which large samples had been measured (girths by Wilmore and Behnke, 1969–1970, skinfolds of unpublished data from Yuhasz, other measurements by Garret and Kennedy, 1971) were used, and the mode of the different anthropometric variables in these populations was calculated. In this case, the mode was chosen because if the mean was used as the final value, the result could be influenced by extreme values. However, the mode is the most repeated value and is not influenced by extreme values.

It should be noted that the *Phantom* method is not representative of any specific population group, as the measurements used to generate the model included a heterogeneous sample composed of people of different ages, from infants to older adults, with different levels of physical activity, different lifestyles and health levels of both sexes. From these data, a model was obtained that cannot be attributed to a specific sex, age or habits. Therefore, through this system, any person can be compared, always bearing in mind that it is not the norm. For all the above, the *Phantom* model is a metaphorical and asexual model, which eliminates bias due to sexual dimorphism, and is therefore suitable for comparing any person of any age.

Firstly, to compare a subject with the *Phantom* model, it should be noted that it proposes an adjustment of the variable according to his/her stretch stature, adjusted to the dimensionality of the variable, as it would not be correct to compare subjects of different stretch statures as they are not proportionally equal. In other words, if two people with a different value in the measurement of the variable and different stretch statures are compared, it will not be possible to know who has proportionally more or less variable, as they are not comparable. This is what allows the *Phantom* method to be applicable to populations with different stretch statures or in the growth phase. For example, if a triceps skinfold of 15 mm is measured in several subjects of different stretch statures, the tallest will have a proportionally smaller skinfold, and the shortest will have a proportionally larger skinfold. However, if one person has a skinfold of 15 mm and another a skinfold of 14 mm, and they are of different stretch statures, it will not be possible to know who has proportionally more skinfold until the variable is adjusted for both cases according to stretch stature.

To make the adjustment of the variable that you want to compare, the value of the analysed variable is multiplied by the stretch stature of the *Phantom* model (170.18 cm) divided by the stretch stature of the subject. If the subject's stretch stature is greater than 170.18 cm (stretch stature of the *Phantom* model), the value after the adjustment of the resulting variable will be smaller than the original value of the variable. On the other hand, if the stretch stature is less than 170.18 cm, the result of the value of that variable will be greater than the initial value of the variable.

In addition, the *Phantom* model reduces all variables to the same scale of dimensionality in order to obtain the same comparison system for all variables, regardless of the dimensions they occupy. This is necessary, as variables that are one-dimensional such as stretch stature, sitting height, arm span, skinfolds, girths, corrected girths, lengths and heights, and breadths and depths, are compared with other two-dimensional variables such as muscle areas, with other three-dimensional ones such as body mass, fat mass, muscle mass, bone mass, or residual mass. Therefore, the *Phantom* model reduces everything to the same dimensional scale in order to compare everything with the same model. Thus, once the variable is adjusted by the stretch stature of the subject, to apply the comparison with the *Phantom* model, the dimensions of the variable must also be adjusted, whether it is a one-dimensional, two-dimensional, or three-dimensional variable.

The mathematical expression of this operation is:

$$\text{Variable adjusted for stretch stature} = v * (170.18/\text{stretch stature (cm)})^{d}$$

Where:

- v = value of the variable to be adjusted.
- d = dimensionality: 1 for stretch stature, sitting height, arm span, skinfolds, girths, corrected girths, lengths and heights, and breadths and depths; 2 for muscle areas; and 3 for body mass, fat mass, muscle mass, bone mass, or residual mass.

Here is an example: Marta is 165 cm tall and has a hips girth of 89 cm. Juan is 180 cm tall and has a hips girth of 95 cm.

For Marta, you have to do: $89 * (170.18/165)^{1} = 91.79$ cm, which is her hips girth adjusted for her stretch stature.
For Juan, you have to do: $95 * (170.18/180)^{1} = 89.81$ cm, which is his hips girth adjusted for his stretch stature.

Therefore, proportionally, Marta has a larger hips girth than Juan.

Here is another example where you have to adjust based on dimensionality: Marta is 165 cm tall and has a body mass of 60 kg. Juan is 180 cm tall and has a body mass of 75 kg.

For Marta, you have to do: $60 * (170.18/165)^{3} = 65.83$ kg, which is her body mass adjusted for her stretch stature, taking into account that the body mass has three dimensions.
For Juan, you have to do: $75 * (170.18/180)^{3} = 63.38$ kg, which is his body mass adjusted for his stretch stature, taking into account that the body mass has three dimensions.

Therefore, proportionally, Marta has more body mass than Juan.

Another issue to consider, with regard to the *Phantom* model, is that it not only considers the population mode for each of the variables, but also the standard deviation. This is because the population is not homogeneous, but has diverse anthropometric characteristics. Therefore, what have to be done in the *Phantom* model, once the variable has been corrected for stretch stature and corrected in terms of dimensionality, is to subtract the mode of the population for the analysed variable, resulting in the comparison of the variable with the mode of the *Phantom* model, which will serve to find if the variable is greater or smaller than this, and it is divided by the standard deviation.

Let's see an example of this:

A person has a waist girth adjusted with the *Phantom* model based on their stretch stature of 67 cm and dimensionality (shown in previous step). The population mode of the *Phantom* model for this variable is 71.91 cm and the deviation is 4.45 cm.

1. The difference in cm between the person's waist girth and that of the population will be calculated. Thus: 67 – 71.91 = – 4.91 cm. That is, this person has a waist 4.91 cm smaller than the population mode.
2. But this can be a lot or a little depending on how homogeneous the population is. Thus, the next step is to find the units of standard deviation that correspond to this difference. In our case: – 4.91 cm/4.45 cm per unit of deviation (standard deviation of the *Phantom*) = – 1.10.

The calculation of the standard deviations that exist between a subject and the population is what the model *Phantom* refers to as the Z index. That is, the *Phantom* model is a mathematical model that serves to find how many deviations a particular subject deviates from the population mode in a variable that has been corrected based on the subject's stretch stature and the dimensionality of the variable. The formula for calculating the Z indices is as follows:

$$Z = ((v^*((170.18/H)^d) - p))/s$$

Where:

s: Standard deviation of the *Phantom* model, relative to the measurement under study.
v: Subject's measurement.
H: Subject's stretch stature.
p: Mode of the variable analysed in the *Phantom* model.
^{d}: Is the exponent. (1) For linear measurements (stretch stature, sitting height, arm span, skinfolds, girths, corrected girths, lengths and heights, breadths and depths); (2) For surface measurements and cross-sectional areas (muscle areas); (3) For mass measurements and volumes (body mass, fat mass, muscle mass, bone mass and residual mass).

To do this, it is necessary to know the modes and standard deviation of the *Phantom* model. These can be found in Table 6.10.

Let's see an example of how to calculate the Z index. An athlete of 180.3 cm for stretch stature and has a leg girth of 39.50 cm:

1. Correct the variable based on the individual's stretch stature and the dimensionality: 39.50 * $(170.18/180.3)^1$ = 39.50 * 0.94 = 37.28.

Table 6.10 Modes and standard deviation of the *Phantom* method

Variable	Mode	Standard deviation
Body mass	64.58	8.60
Height	170.18	6.29
Sitting height	89.92	4.50
Arm span	172.35	7.41
Triceps skinfold	15.40	4.47
Subscapular skinfold	17.20	5.07
Biceps skinfold	8.00	2.00
Iliac crest skinfold	22.40	6.80
Supraspinale skinfold	15.40	4.47
Abdominal skinfold	25.40	7.78
Thigh skinfold	27.00	8.33
Calf skinfold	16.00	4.67
Head girth	56.00	1.44
Neck girth	34.91	1.73
Arm relaxed girth	26.89	2.33
Arm flexed and tensed girth	29.41	2.37
Forearm girth	25.13	1.41
Wrist girth	16.35	0.72
Chest girth	87.86	5.18
Waist girth	71.91	4.45
Hips girth	94.67	5.58
Thigh 1 cm gluteal girth	55.82	4.23
Thigh middle girth	53.20	4.56
Calf girth	35.25	2.30
Ankle girth	21.71	1.33
Arm corrected girth	22.05	1.91
Chest corrected girth	82.46	4.86
Thigh corrected girth	47.34	3.59
Calf corrected girth	30.22	1.97
Acromiale-Radiale length	32.53	1.77
Radiale-Stylion length	24.57	1.37
Midstylion-Dactylion length	18.85	0.85
Ilioespinale height	94.11	4.71
Trochanterion height	86.40	4.32
Trochanterion-Tibiale laterale length	41.37	2.48

(continued)

Table 6.10 (continued)

Variable	Mode	Standard deviation
Tibiale laterale height	45.20	2.67
Foot length	25.50	1.16
Tibiale mediale-Sphyrion tibiale length	36.81	2.10
Biacromial breadth	38.04	1.92
Biiliocristal breadth	28.84	1.75
Transverse chest breadth	27.92	1.74
Antero-posterior chest depth	17.50	1.38
Humerus breadth	6.48	0.35
Bi-styloid breadth	5.21	0.28
Femur breadth	9.52	0.48
Bimalleolar breadth	6.68	0.37
Sum of six skinfolds	116.41	34.79
Lipid mass	12.13	3.25
Adipose mass	25.60	5.85
Muscle mass	24.50	5.40
Bone mass	10.49	1.57
Residual mass	6.10	1.24

2. Subtract the value of the mode of the *Phantom* model for that variable, in this case it is 35.25 cm. So: 37.28 − 35.25 = 2.03.
3. Calculate the standard deviation units that correspond to the difference based on the standard deviation of the *Phantom* model for that variable, in this case, 2.30 cm. Therefore: 2.03/2.30 = 0.88.

Therefore, the athlete has a leg girth 0.88 standard deviation units greater than that of the *Phantom* model.

Following this method, if a subject has a Z index equal to 0, it means that they are proportionally the same as the mode of the *Phantom* model for that particular variable. If the Z index is positive, it means that the size-adjusted variable is proportionally larger than that of the *Phantom* model. If the Z index is negative, it means that the size-adjusted variable is smaller than that of the *Phantom* model.

Applying the notions of statistics according to a normal distribution as per the Gaussian bell curve, if a subject is found within a unit of deviation, with respect to the *Phantom* model or another person or population, it is considered that there are no differences. If the subject is found between one and two deviations, it will be considered that this subject has a tendency to be different from the *Phantom* model or the subject or population with whom they are being compared. And if the subject is found more than two deviations up or down, it can be considered that this subject is significantly different from the *Phantom* model or to the subject

Table 6.11 Interpretation of *Phantom* scores

Phantom score value	Interpretation
< − 2	Subject whose height-adjusted variable is significantly lower than the Phantom (population mode) or the group/subject to which he/she is being compared
− 2 to − 1	Subject whose size-adjusted variable has a tendency to be lower than the Phantom (population mode) or the group/subject to which he/she is being compared
− 1 to + 1	Subject whose size-adjusted variable is similar to the Phantom (population mode) or the group/subject to which he/she is being compared
+ 1 to + 2	Subject whose size-adjusted variable has a tendency to be higher than Phantom (population mode) or the group/subject to which he/she is being compared
> +2	Subject whose height-adjusted variable is significantly higher than the Phantom (population mode) or the group/subject to which he/she is being compared

or population with whom they are being compared. This means that, for example, if a 100 m sprinter has a Z score of + 2 for the corrected leg girth, and his/her training group has a Z score of + 1.5 for said girth, the runner has a significantly higher value than the *Phantom* model, but similar to his/her training group in the corrected leg girth. On the other hand, if the Z value of the corrected leg girth of another teammate is + 3.6, this subject tends to have more corrected leg girth than the previous runner (between 1 and 2 units of difference in the Z value), and significantly more corrected leg girth than his/her training group and that of the *Phantom* model (more than 2 units of difference in the Z value). The interpretation of the values of the *Phantom* model can be found in Table 6.11.

Some of the fields in which the *Phantom* model strategy has been applied are:

- Analysis of the changes of anthropometric variables in growing population. In this population, absolute variables are not comparable as they are conditioned by the changes in dimensionality that occur when growing. A good solution to this is the calculation of Z values to analyse the changes of the growing population, as it relativises the variables according to stretch stature. This is especially important during puberty, as this is when most physical changes occur in a shorter period of time. Thus, it is possible that when comparing the absolute variables measured in an individual, no changes will be found in them, although there may be a change in the proportionality of the individual, and this will not be possible to find if the *Phantom* method is not applied to this analysis. For example, if the subject has the same skinfold and has the same girth, but the stretch stature has increased by one centimetre, proportionally, the value of these measurements is lower. Therefore, the use of the *Phantom* model in growing populations is very interesting, as it allows following the growth proportionally and without stretch stature and growth being contaminating variables when comparing the values obtained.
- Comparison of the measurements of an athlete or group of athletes with the measurements of a reference athlete or group of athletes, such as elite athletes.

This will allow us to find in which variables our athlete tends to have a difference with the reference group or is significantly different from the reference group, so that in case the variable is modifiable and represents a competitive disadvantage, we can proceed to make the changes in training/diet that lead to its modification in the desired direction.

- Comparison of anthropometric variables within the same individual. By adjusting all variables to the same dimension and scale, the *Phantom* model allows us to analyse the amount of muscle development (corrected girths) and bone (breadths) that exists in a certain area. A difference in favour of muscle development could mean that the subject has more power and acceleration capacity as there is less mass to move in the movements in which the segment is involved, as is the case with a basketball shot for the upper limb, a jump for the lower limb. Now, this also involves a higher risk of injury, as the muscle traction could be excessive for the bone support that exists, affecting both the bone itself, as well as the muscle and tendon, so it is a matter to be taken into account in sports planning.

6.4 Questionnaire

1. Proportionality refers to:
   (a) It is a branch of knowledge that analyses the relationship between anthropometric measurements to understand their relative size.
   (b) It has different fields of application, such as ergonomics or sports performance.
   (c) It is a branch of knowledge that analyses the relationship of the whole body with some reference to understand its relative size.
   (d) All are true.
2. Regarding the application of proportionality to sports performance:
   (a) In elite athletes of the same discipline or position, similarity in anthropometric proportions can be observed.
   (b) In elite athletes of the same discipline or position, there is a great heterogeneity in terms of anthropometric proportions.
   (c) Proportionality has no evidence in relation to sports performance.
   (d) There are no theories about proportionality and sports performance.
3. Regarding body indices, indicate the false one:
   (a) Indices are expressed as a percentage.
   (b) Relative measurements, indices, and ponderal indices are three types of body indices.
   (c) To calculate an index, the larger measurement is always divided by the smaller one.
   (d) With indices, it can be verified whether a measurement is proportionally large or small as compared to another.
4. The relative sitting height:
   (a) Relates the length of the upper and lower limb.

   (b) Relates sitting height and stretch stature.
   (c) Relates body mass and stretch stature.
   (d) Relates the length of the lower limb with stretch stature.
5. When the value of the acromial-iliac index is between 70 and 74.9% in men, it can be referred to as:
   (a) Rectangular trunk.
   (b) Trapezoidal trunk.
   (c) Intermediate trunk.
   (d) None of the above.
6. The waist-hip index has been mainly related to:
   (a) Better sports performance.
   (b) It has no relation with any other variable.
   (c) Greater ergonomics.
   (d) Risk of suffering metabolic diseases.
7. For the fat distribution index, indicate the false one:
   (a) It is usually the same in men and women.
   (b) The accumulation of fat in the trunk provides stability in most sports.
   (c) If the result is lower, it indicates a tendency to accumulate fat in the trunk.
   (d) Women tend to have a greater accumulation of fat in the legs.
8. Regarding proportionality and sports performance:
   (a) A greater relative length of the upper limb favours performance in sports such as volleyball, handball, or basketball.
   (b) Performance in weightlifting is favoured by long limbs.
   (c) A short lower limb favours running.
   (d) None are true.
9. Regarding BMI:
   (a) It is a body mass index that relates stretch stature to body mass.
   (b) Traditionally, it has been related to health parameters.
   (c) It has limitations, such as comparing variables of different dimensions without properly adjusting them.
   (d) All of the above are true.
10. Regarding the Phantom model, indicate the false one:
   (a) It is a model that allows the comparison of individuals by relativising measurements based on stretch stature.
   (b) It allows us to find if a variable is proportionally higher or lower than the model.
   (c) There is a different model for men and women.
   (d) It allows us to analyse the differences between two individuals.

Answers:

1.d, 2.a, 3.c, 4.b, 5.c, 6.d, 7.a, 8.a, 9.d, 10.c

Bibliography

Esparza-Ros F., Vaquero-Cristóbal R., & Marfell-Jones M. (2019). *International protocol for anthropometric assessment*. International Society for the Advancement of Kinanthropometry.

Norton, K., & Olds, T. (1996). *Anthropometrica.* New South Wales Press.

Ross, W. D., & Kerr, D. A. (1991). Fractionation of body mass: A new method for use in clinical nutrition and sports medicine. *Apunts. Medicina de l´Esport, 18*(1), 175–187.

Ross, W. D., & Wilson, N. C. (1974). A stratagem for proportional growth assessment. *Acta Paediatrica Belgica, 28*, 169–182.

Analysis of the Somatotype Through Anthropometric Assessment

7

Abstract

This chapter contains information about the definition of the somatotype as a method to quantify the shape and composition of the human body, providing a quantitative summary of the current physique. It specifies which methods and formulas are used to calculate the three components of the somatotype: endomorphy (adiposity), mesomorphy (muscular and bone development), and ectomorphy (thinness). It then specifies how to classify the somatotype into thirteen established categories and interpret them, and shows how to calculate the X and Y coordinates of the somatopoint to graphically represent the somatotype on a somatochart. Information is included on how to calculate the average somatotype of a group, how to calculate the differences in the somatotype between a subject and a group, how to calculate the homogeneity of the somatotype within a group, and how to calculate the differences in the somatotype between one group and another. Finally, the issues to be considered in the application and interpretation of the somatotype are specified.

Keywords

Endomorphy • Mesomorphy • Ectomorphy • Somatopoint • Somatochart • Anthropometric method • Photoscopic method

7.1 Definition

The somatotype is a method of quantifying the shape and current composition of the human body that provides a quantitative summary of the physique as a unified whole at the time it is studied. The somatotype is phenotypic, so both genetics and the environmental conditions and lifestyle habits acquired by the person are important.

© The Author(s), under exclusive license to Springer Nature Switzerland AG 2025

F. Esparza-Ros and R. Vaquero-Cristóbal, *Anthropometry*,
https://doi.org/10.1007/978-3-031-77535-2_7

To express the somatotype, three components are calculated, which are always presented in the same order (X-Y-Z). Although the separation between the components is made with a hyphen (-), it does not represent a negative value since the numbers of the somatotype are always positive and greater than zero. Each component represents:

- Endomorphy (X): The first component. It refers to relative adiposity. Accumulation of "fat".
- Mesomorphy (Y): The second component. It refers to relative musculoskeletal magnitude. Muscle and bone development.
- Ectomorphy (Z): The third component. It represents relative linearity or thinness. Predominance of longitudinal measurements over transverse ones.

As can be observed, while endomorphy and mesomorphy refer to the subject's body composition (fat, muscle and bone), the ectomorphy variable refers more to shape. In addition, an increase in the endomorphic and/or mesomorphic components leads to a decrease in ectomorphy, while a decrease in endomorphy or mesomorphy results in an increase in ectomorphy.

The most relevant aspect of the somatotype is that it provides information about the unique combination of three aspects of the physique in the primary components (fat, muscle and linearity) through a single expression of three numbers. However, the main drawback of the somatotype is that it describes the physique in general, without addressing the specific dimensions of the body, so it is unknown how the distribution of fat, muscle, bone or linearity occurs in the subject's body. To solve this problem, within the anthropometric method, there are other measures such as the skinfold sums and the skinfold profile, corrected girths and transverse muscle areas, and/or the Z indices of the *Phantom* that allow us to know the differences in the specific dimensions of these components in order to be able to understand the evolution of adiposity and musculoskeletal development in a specific body area, which is especially relevant in the sports field.

7.2 Calculation of the Somatotype

There are two methods for calculating the somatotype: the photoscopic method and the anthropometric method:

- Photoscopic method

The photoscopic method involves taking photographs of the subject (from the front, both sides and from the back) with little or no clothing. To carry out the measurement, you need: a good quality camera, a tripod located 5.8 m from the subject, minimal clothing, and a room equipped with grids located behind the subject to allow subsequent measurements on the photographs to calculate the somatotype. This method is currently in disuse for several reasons: it is a fairly invasive system with the subject to be evaluated; it does not allow for a general field evaluation; and it only allows for the calculation of the somatotype, so the limitations of this method cannot be resolved by combining and interpreting it with other methods. For all these reasons, this method is practically in disuse today.

- Anthropometric method

For the calculation of the somatotype using anthropometry, the Heath-Carter method is used. The anthropometric method is currently the most utilized method for calculating the somatotype due to the advantages it presents over the photoscopic method, such as adaptability to both field and laboratory measurements in different spaces, for its ability to provide information beyond the somatotype with the anthropometric measurements made, because it requires little equipment and few calculations, for being an "easy" measurement, and that it allows evaluating the subjects with the minimum amount of clothing. Lastly, as long as the issues established in the topic of ethics and proxemics are taken into account, it is a less invasive method for the subject evaluated.

Not in vain, for the calculation of the somatotype, only ten measurements are needed:

- Basic measurements: body mass and stretch stature.
- Triceps, subscapular, supraspinal and calf skinfolds.
- Arm flexed and tensed, and calf girths.
- Humerus and femur breadths.

Next, Table 7.1 shows the variables that are entered in the calculation of each of the components of the somatotype, and how their change modifies this component.

The inclusion of stretch stature in both the endomorphic and mesomorphic component, maintaining the differences in the way it is included in each of them, is a strong point of the somatotype, as it allows relativizing adiposity or musculoskeletal mass according to the stretch stature of the subject.

- Anthropometric method + Photoscopic method

The inclusion of the two methods in parallel is considered the gold standard for the calculation of the somatotype. However, the difficulties presented in the implementation of the photoscopic method make this not a frequently used approach.

Table 7.1 Variation of the somatotype components as a function of anthropometric variables assessed

	Endomorphy	Mesomorphy	Ectomorphy
Height	If it increases, endomorphy decreases	If it increases, mesomorphy decreases	If it increases, ectomorphy increases
Body mass			If it increases, ectomorphy decreases
Triceps skinfold	If it increases, endomorphy increases	If it increases, mesomorphy decreases	
Subscapular skinfold	If it increases, endomorphy increases		
Supraspinal skinfold	If it increases, endomorphy increases		
Leg skinfold		If it increases, mesomorphy decreases	
Arm flexed and tensed girth		If it increases, mesomorphy increases	
Calf girth		If it increases, mesomorphy increases	
Humerus breadth		If it increases, mesomorphy increases	
Femur breadth		If it increases, mesomorphy increases	

7.2.1 Methods for Calculating the Somatotype Using the Anthropometric Method

The calculation of the somatotype through anthropometric measurements can be carried out using a pro forma template sheet of values or by applying formulas. Regarding the use of the sheet, this method consists of, once the anthropometric assessment of the ten specified variables has been carried out, performing a series of standardised steps on a template for the calculation of the somatotype. However, this method has some disadvantages, such as the time required to calculate the somatotype of each component, or the fact that the numbers it reports are whole or half (X.0 or X.5). Therefore, its scale is less discriminatory than when the somatotype is calculated using formulas.

For all the above, the anthropometric method of applying formulas is the most commonly utilized method for calculating the somatotype. The formulas to apply are as follows:

- Calculation of the endomorphic component

The formula to apply for the calculation of this component is:

$$\begin{aligned} Endomorphy = & -0.7182 + 0.1451 * Xc \\ & - 0.00068 * Xc^2 + 0.0000014 * Xc^3 \end{aligned}$$

where:

- X: Σ Triceps skinfold (mm) + Subscapular skinfold (mm) + Supraspinal skinfold (mm).
- Corrected X (Xc): Value of “X” corrected based on stretch stature of the subject and the stretch stature of the Phantom model: = X * (170.18/Stretch stature (cm)).

This formula yields values for endomorphy between ½ and 16, with normal values mostly ranging between 1 and 8.

- Calculation of the mesomorphic component.

The formula to apply for the calculation of this component is:

$$\begin{aligned} Mesomorphy = & \ 0.858 * \textit{Humerus breadth}\,(\text{cm}) + 0.601 * \textit{Femur breadth}\,(\text{cm}) \\ & + 0.188 * \textit{Arm corrected girth}\,(\text{cm}) + 0.161 * \textit{Calf corrected girth}\,(\text{cm}) \\ & - 0.131 * \textit{Height}\,(\text{cm}) + 4.55 \end{aligned}$$

where:

- Corrected arm girth = Arm flexed and tensed girth (cm) − Triceps skinfold (cm).
- Corrected calf girth = Calf girth (cm) − Calf skinfold (cm).

This formula yields values for mesomorphy between ½ and 12, with normal values mostly between 1 and 7.

- Calculation of the ectomorphic component.

To calculate this component, the specific ponderal index of the somatotype must first be calculated:

$$\textit{Ponderal index} = \frac{\textit{Height}\,(\text{cm})}{\sqrt[3]{\textit{Body mass}\,(\text{kg})}}$$

Once the ponderal index for the somatotype has been calculated, a specific formula is applied depending on the result of the ponderal index:

If ponderal index $\geq$ 40.75 $\rightarrow$ Ectomorphy = (ponderal index * 0.732) − 28.58.
If ponderal index < 40.75 and > 38.28 $\rightarrow$ Ectomorphy = (ponderal index * 0.463) − 17.63.
If ponderal index $\leq$ 38.28 $\rightarrow$ Ectomorphy = 0.1 (Fixed value).

This formula yields values for ectomorphy between 0.1 and 10, with normal values mostly between 0.1 and 7.

7.3 Aspects to Consider in the Calculation and Interpretation of the Somatotype

There are a number of considerations to bear in mind in the calculation and interpretation of the somatotype:

- In the interpretation of the reported results, it is generally interpreted that when the value of a component is less than 3 it is considered low, when the value lies between 3.1 and 5, it is considered a moderate value, when the value is between 5.1 and 7, it is considered high, and when the value is greater than 7.1 the component is extremely high.
- If the calculation for any component is zero or a negative number, a value of 0.1 is assigned, as this cannot be true by definition. However, before doing this, it must be verified that there has been no error in the data (for example, in the unit of measuring the variables or the placement of the variables in the proforma sheet).
- It is rare to find an endomorphy and mesomorphy of less than 1. In ectomorphy, this happens more frequently.
- Certain somatotype classifications are not biologically possible (for example, 2-2-2 or 7-8-7), as there are components that are opposing, so a higher value of it (endomorphy or mesomorphy) leads to a lower value of another component (ectomorphy).
- Generally, if endomorphy and mesomorphy are high, ectomorphy is low. These parameters in the field of sport are common in combat sports or body-to-body contact sports. If ectomorphy is high, endomorphy and mesomorphy are low. These parameters in the field of sport are common in endurance sports, jumping sports, or in those where the mobility of one's own body mass is a handicap for sports performance.

7.4 Limitations in the Calculation of the Somatotype

The variables that each component of the somatotype includes are not exempt from limitations. The main ones are:

- Endomorphy: The somatotype does not include any lower limb skinfold for the calculation of this component, with this being a considerable error.
- Mesomorphy: The triceps and calf skinfolds are used for the calculation of the corrected arm and calf girths, respectively, in order to estimate the muscle component. But this is done incorrectly from a mathematical point of view, when not introducing "π" in the formula. Thus, while the correct formula for the calculation of the corrected girths is girth (cm) $- \pi$ * skinfold (cm), the formula used for the calculation of the girths in the somatotype is girth (cm) – skinfold (cm). It must also be added that the corrected arm girth is not calculated with the arm relaxed girth, as it should be done, as it is the girth that is taken in the same place as the skinfold, but with the arm flexed and tensed girth which is more distal to the place where the skinfold is measured.
- Ectomorphy: The calculation of this component is done by calculating the ponderal index, an index that relates body mass and stretch stature. However, the formula used is not correct. Because, instead of dividing the body mass by the stretch stature cubed, a formula classically used for the calculation of the ponderal index (Ponderal Index = body mass (g) * 100/stretch stature (cm)^3), it divides the stretch stature by the cube root of the body mass (Ponderal Index in the somatotype = stretch stature (cm)/$\sqrt[3]{}$ body mass (kg)), which makes them report completely different results. In spite of this, it maintains dimensionality.

7.5 The Somatochart

The somatotype is graphically represented in the triangle by Franz Reuleaux, better known as somatochart. This is a two-dimensional graphic scheme with two axes (X, Y) in which the somatotype is represented in a single point called the somatopoint. The resulting "X" and "Y" coordinates are the result of independently adding the projections (vectors) on the "X" and "Y" axes of the three components of the somatotype. It should be noted that in the somatochart, the axes are not proportional, with the vertical unit (Y) being greater than the horizontal (X) one in order to represent a three-dimensional image in only two dimensions. The relationship is $Y = X/\sqrt{3}$.

To calculate the somatopoint, the following formulas must be applied:

- X = ectomorphy – endomorphy.
- Y = 2 * mesomorphy – (ectomorphy + endomorphy).

Next, an example of the calculation of the somatopoint from the somatotype is presented. In a subject who presents a somatotype (3-4-2), the coordinates on the

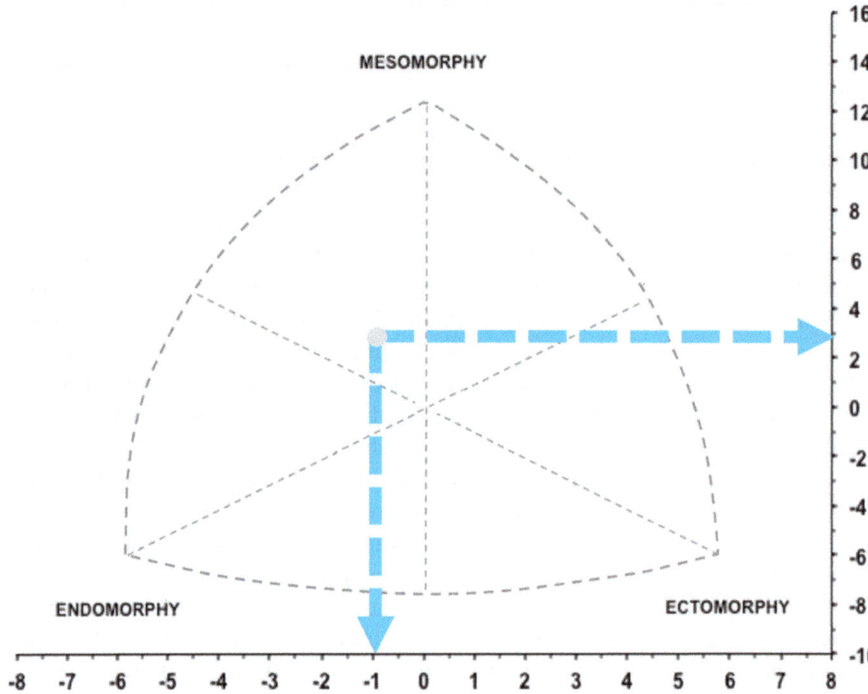

Fig. 7.1 Example of somatotype representation on the somatochart

somatochart will be: X = 2 − 3 = − 1; Y = 2 * 4 − (3 + 2) = 8 − 5 = 3 (Fig. 7.1).

The vertices of the somatochart are as follows (Fig. 7.2):

- X = 0, Y = 12 (0, 12). Corresponding somatotype: 1-7-1 Subject with great mesomorphic development.
- X = − 6, Y = − 6 (− 6, − 6). Corresponding somatotype: 7-1-1 Subject with great endomorphic development.
- X = 6, Y = − 6 (6, − 6). Corresponding somatotype: 1-1-7 Subject with great ectomorphic development.

The behaviour of the somatopoint on the somatochart is as follows:

- A shift to the right indicates that ectomorphy is greater than endomorphy. Therefore, if the somatopoint shifts to the right, it may be due to an increase in ectomorphy or a decrease in endomorphy.

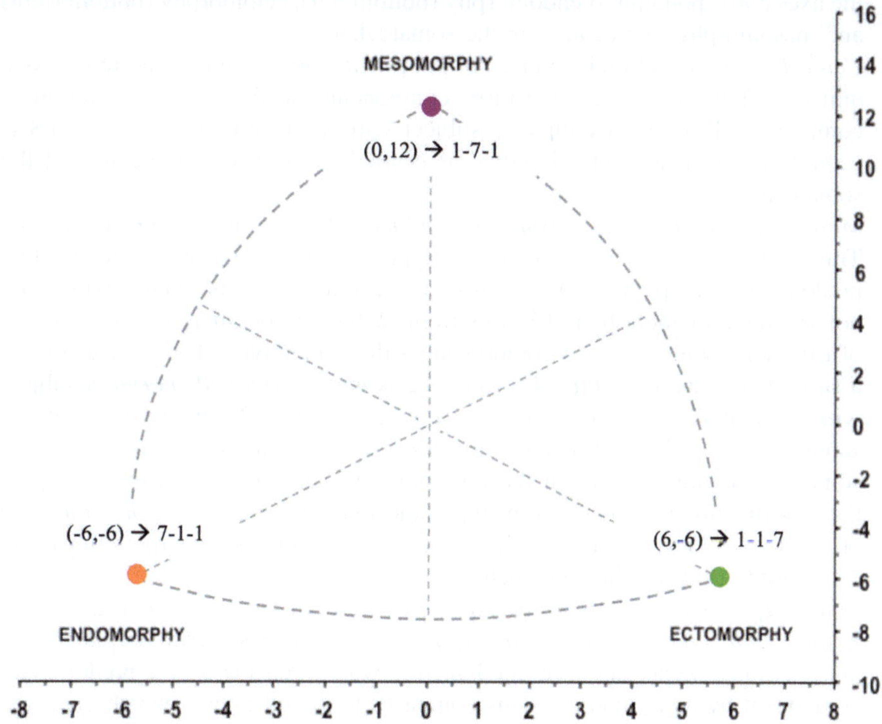

Fig. 7.2 Vertices of the somatochart and somatopoints

- A shift to the left indicates that endomorphy is greater than ectomorphy. Therefore, if the somatopoint shifts to the left it may be due to an increase in endomorphy or a decrease in ectomorphy.
- The upward shift of the somatopoint indicates an increase in mesomorphy.

7.6 Classification of the Somatotype

The somatotype classification system allows it to be classified into:

- *Balanced mesomorph, Balanced endomorph or Balanced ectomorph*: when one of the components is greater, and the other two components do not differ from each other by more than 0.5 units. The predominant component is the one that gives the name to the classification. The term balanced refers to there being no differences of more than 0.5 units between the other two components. Thus, for example, a subject with a somatotype $5 - 3 - 2.8$ is a *balanced endomorph*. The *balanced* somatotypes correspond to the somatopoints located at the vertices of the axes corresponding to endomorphy (bottom left), ectomorphy (bottom right) and mesomorphy (top centre) on the somatochart.

- *Central*: A classification is referred to as *central* when there is no more than one unit of difference between the three components, so there is no predominant component. Thus, for example, a subject with a somatotype 4 – 4 – 3.8 is central. The somatopoints classified as *central* are located in the centre of the somatochart.
- *Mesomorph-ectomorph*, *mesomorph-endomorph* or *endomorph-ectomorph*: This is the name given to the somatotype classification when there are two predominant components (which give the classification its name), which are not separated by more than 0.5 units from each other, but there is at least 1 unit of difference with the third component of the somatotype. Thus, for example, a subject with a somatotype 4 – 3.6 – 2 is *mesomorph-endomorph*, a subject with a somatotype 1 – 4 – 3.6 is *mesomorph-ectomorph*, and a subject with a somatotype 3 – 1 – 2.6 is *endomorph-ectomorph.* On the somatochart, these somatopoints are arranged at the midpoint between the two vertices that give the classification its name. For example, the somatotype *mesomorph-ectomorph* (1 – 4 – 3.6) is located at the midpoint between mesomorphy (top) and ectomorphy (left) on the somatochart.
- *Endomorphic mesomorph*, *Ectomorphic mesomorph*, *Mesomorphic endomorph*, *Ectomorphic endomorph*, *Mesomorphic ectomorph* and *Endomorphic ectomorph*: Somatotypes are classified in this way when there is a predominant component by more than 0.5 units compared to the other two (which gives the second name of the classification), but there is more than 0.5 units between the other two components, i.e., there is a second dominant component (which gives the first name of the classification). Thus, for example, a subject with a somatotype 3.3 – 5 – 2 is *endomorphic mesomorph*; a subject with a somatotype 2 – 5 – 3.3 is *ectomorphic mesomorph*; a subject with a somatotype 5 – 3.3 – 2 is *mesomorphic endomorph*; a subject with a somatotype 5 – 2 – 3.3 is *ectomorphic endomorph;* a subject with a somatotype 2 – 3.3 – 5 is *mesomorphic ectomorph*; and a subject with a somatotype 3.3 – 2 – 5 is *endomorphic ectomorph.* When these subjects are represented on the somatochart, they are found in the areas located between the two predominant components, closer to the predominant component, but not reaching the axis.

7.7 Analysis of the Somatotype

This allows us to discover if an individual is changing significantly, if they differ from a group, or if there is homogeneity within a group. For this, an individual analysis or a group analysis can be carried out, both with the X and Y coordinates, as well as with the components (endomorphy, mesomorphy, and ectomorphy). Next, we will see the options that the analysis of the somatotype offers:

7.7.1 Calculation of the Mean Somatotype of a Group

It is used to find the average somatotype of a group or population. For the calculation of the average somatotype of the group, the calculation of the mean somatotype (MS) is used. The formula averages each of the components of the somatotype of the individuals who make up that group. The formula to apply is as follows:

$$\text{Mean somatotype} = \left[\frac{\sum Endomorphy}{n}; \frac{\sum Mesomorphy}{n}; \frac{\sum Ectomorphy}{n}\right]$$

where:

- $\sum$ Endomorphy $_n$: Sum of the endomorphic component of all the subjects in the group.
- $\sum$ Mesomorphy $_n$: Sum of the mesomorphic component of all the subjects in the group.
- $\sum$ Ectomorphy $_n$: Sum of the ectomorphic component of all the subjects in the group.
- n: number of subjects in the group.

Below is an example of how to calculate the mean somatotype of a group. The group consists of seven subjects:

A: 1.4 – 7.7 – 1.1
B: 1.5 – 5.6 – 2.0
C: 2.1 – 8.0 – 0.8
D: 2.0 – 5.2 – 2.9
E: 1.5 – 5.2 – 3.3
F: 1.7 – 5.5 – 2.3
G: 1.6 – 5.8 – 2.8

The calculation operation is as follows:

$$\text{Endomorphy mean} = \frac{(1.4 + 1.5 + 2.1 + 2.0 + 1.5 + 1.7 + 1.6)}{7} = 1.7$$

$$\text{Mesomorphy mean} = \frac{(7.7 + 5.6 + 8.0 + 5.2 + 5.2 + 5.5 + 5.8)}{7} = 6.1$$

$$\text{Ectomorphy mean} = \frac{(1.1 + 2.0 + 0.8 + 2.9 + 3.3 + 2.3 + 2.8)}{7} = 2.2$$

Therefore, the average somatotype of this group is: 1.7 – 6.1 – 2.2.

7.7.2 Calculation of the Differences in the Somatotype Between a Subject and a Group

The analysis of the calculation of the differences between a subject and a group allows us to find to what extent the subject we are analysing resembles or not the group. Thus, if we find that the subject is different from the group, we can, if necessary, adjust the somatotype of the individual to that of the group.

This can be done by calculating the Somatotype Dispersion Distance (SDD), based on the X and Y coordinates, or the somatotype attitudinal distance (SAD), based on the components (endomorphy, mesomorphy, ectomorphy).

7.7.2.1 Somatotype Dispersion Distance (SDD)

Based on the somatopoint, it serves to compare an individual (X_1, Y_1) with a group (X_2, Y_2). What is done is to calculate the difference between two points represented in a vector system, calculating the distance from one point to another in X and Y.

$$\text{Somatotype dispersion distance (SDD)} = \sqrt{3 * (X_1 - X_2)^2 + (Y_1 - Y_2)^2}$$

where:

- X_1: Value of the coordinate on the X axis of the somatotype chart of the subject to be compared.
- X_2: Average of the group with which the subject is compared for the value of the X axis of the somatotype chart.
- Y_1: Value of the coordinate on the Y axis of the somatotype chart of the subject to be compared.
- Y_2: Average of the group with which the subject is compared for the value of the Y axis of the somatotype chart.

The result is a figure. If $SDD \geq 2$, the subject's somatotype is significantly different from that of the group. From here, it will be necessary to analyse whether a nutritional and training intervention is needed to adjust their somatotype to that of the group.

In order to make this adjustment, it is important to note that the main disadvantage of the SDD is that it does not determine how the individual really differs from the reference, nor how to act to bring them closer to the average. For this reason, the first thing that is done when $SDD \geq 2$ is to compare the endomorphy. If this is greater than that of the reference group, the volume of training can be increased and/or a negative energy balance can be created through diet. If the subject's endomorphy is less than that of the group, an analysis will be performed to find whether this situation is a handicap; if it does not affect the proposed objectives, no adjustments will be made. In this sense, it is a mistake to think that presenting less endomorphy than the reference group means that the solution is to increase this component, as it will be a burden in terms of sports performance and general health.

Once the endomorphy comparison has been made, the mesomorphy must be compared. If the subject presents a lower mesomorphy than the group, in general, an increase in muscle mass should be sought with appropriate physical exercise, accompanied by a diet adjustment. However, if the athlete presents a higher mesomorphy than the group, it should not be automatically corrected unless there is a reason to do so, as could happen when it would be a competitive disadvantage.

Below is an example of the above. A long jumper has a somatotype of 1.7 – 6.1 – 2.0 (0.3; 8.5). The average somatotype of elite long jumpers in the country is 1.4 – 7.7 – 1.1 (– 0.3; 12.9).

$$\text{Somatotype dispersion distance (SDD)} = \sqrt{3 * (0.3 - (-0.3)^2 + (8.5 - 12.9)^2}$$
$$= \sqrt{3 * (0.6)^2 + (4.4)^2} = \sqrt{3 * 0.36 + 19.36}$$
$$= \sqrt{1.08 + 19.36} = \sqrt{20.44} = 4.52$$

Therefore, there are significant differences between the jumper and the reference because 4.52 > 2. Regarding the adjustments to be made, upon comparing the endomorphy of the athlete and the group, it is found that it should be reduced. When comparing the mesomorphy, it is found that it should be increased. Therefore, the adjustments to be made are to decrease the endomorphy and increase the mesomorphy.

7.7.2.2 Somatotype Attitudinal Distance (SAD)

It is used to compare the three components of the subject's somatotype (I_2, II_2, III_2) with the group (I_1, II_1, III_1). The formula to apply for its calculation is:

$$\text{Somatotype attitudinal distance (SAD)} = \sqrt{(I_1 - I_2)^2 + (II_1 - II_2)^2 + (III_1 - III_2)^2}$$

where:

- I_1: Endomorphic component of the group.
- II_1: Mesomorphic component of the group.
- III_1: Ectomorphic component of the group.
- I_2: Endomorphic component of the subject.
- II_2: Mesomorphic component of the subject.
- III_2: Ectomorphic component of the subject.

The main limitation of the SAD is that it reports a value referring to the difference in the individual's somatotype as compared to the group, without there being cut-off points to aid with its interpretation.

Next, the calculation of the SAD with the previous data is presented (a long jumper has a somatotype of 1.7 – 6.1 – 2.0. The average somatotype of the country's elite long jumpers is 1.4 – 7.7 – 1.1).

$$\begin{aligned}\text{Somatotype attitudinal distance (SAD)} &= \sqrt{(1.4-1.7)^2+(7.7-6.1)^2+(1.1-2.0)^2}\\ &= \sqrt{(-0.3)^2+(1.6)^2+(-0.9)^2}\\ &= \sqrt{0.09+2.56+0.81}\\ &= \sqrt{3.46}=1.86\end{aligned}$$

Therefore, the SAD between the jumper and the group is 1.86 (without any cut-off points to interpret this result).

7.7.3 Calculation of the Homogeneity of the Somatotype Within a Group

This issue is very important in the sports field, because if a group is not homogeneous, presenting certain variables will not be as decisive for performance. However, if the group is very homogeneous in the variables that provide a competitive advantage for the group of athletes, it will be necessary to present similar values in those variables to those of the group, to have a higher probability of performing in sports terms.

To calculate the homogeneity based on the X and Y coordinates, the somatotype dispersion mean (SDM) can be used; and by using the components of the somatotype (endomorphy, mesomorphy, ectomorphy), the somatotype attitudinal mean (SAM) can be calculated.

7.7.3.1 Somatotype Dispersion Mean (SDM)

This method involves calculating the average of the somatotype dispersion distances (SDD) of each of the individuals that make up the group using the somatotype coordinates approach. For this, the group's average is needed and knowing how much difference there is between each individual and the group's average. The formula to apply is:

$$\text{Somatotype dispersion mean (SDM)} = \frac{\Sigma SDD}{n}$$

where:

- SDD: somatotype dispersion distances of each of the individuals that make up the group.
- n: number of individuals that make up the group.

The result is a figure. If SDM ≥ 2, the differences are significant within the group, so the sample is not homogeneous.

Below is an example of the application of this. There are seven athletes who belong to the same group:

A: 1.4 – 7.7 – 1.1 (– 0.3, 12.9)
B: 1.5 – 5.6 – 2.0 (0.5, 7.7)
C: 2.1 – 8.0 – 0.8 (– 1.3, 13.1)
D: 2.0 – 5.2 – 2.9 (0.9, 5.5)
E: 1.5 – 5.2 – 3.3 (1.8, 5.6)
F: 1.7 – 5.5 – 2.3 (0.6, 7.0)
G: 1.6 – 5.8 – 2.8 (1.2, 7.2)

The first thing is to calculate the SDD with the previous example shown. In this case:

A: SDD = 4.67
B: SDD = 0.73
C: SDD = 5.60
D: SDD = 3.02
E: SDD = 3.63
F: SDD = 1.44
G: SDD = 1.74

And what remains is to calculate the SDM:

$$\begin{aligned}&\text{Somatotype dispersion mean (SDM)}\\&=\frac{4.67+0.73+5.60+3.02+3.63+1.44+1.74}{7}\\&=2.89\end{aligned}$$

As the result is > 2, it can be said that the sample is not statistically homogeneous, in other words, the group presents a high heterogeneity in its somatotype.

7.7.3.2 Somatotype Attitudinal Mean (SAM)

This method consists of calculating the somatotype attitudinal distance (SAD) of each of the individuals that form the group using the components of the somatotype approach. For this, the group's average is needed, as well as how much difference there is between each individual as compared to the group's average. The formula to apply is:

$$Somatotype\ attitudinal\ mean\ (SAM) = \frac{\Sigma SAD}{n}$$

where:

- SAD: somatotype attitudinal distance.
- n: number of participants.

The higher the value of the somatotype attitudinal mean, the less homogeneous the group is, but there is no cut-off value to establish significant differences.

Below is an example of the application of this. It starts with the same group as in the previous case:

A: 1.4 – 7.7 – 1.1
B: 1.5 – 5.6 – 2.0
C: 2.1 – 8.0 – 0.8
D: 2.0 – 5.2 – 2.9
E: 1.5 – 5.2 – 3.3
F: 1.7 – 5.5 – 2.3
G: 1.6 – 5.8 – 2.8

The first thing is to calculate the SAD with the previous example shown. In this case:

A: SAD = 1.91
B: SAD = 0.60
C: SAD = 2.35
D: SAD = 1.23
E: SAD = 1.48
F: SAD = 0.66
G: SAD = 0.72

And what remains is to calculate the SAM:

$$\begin{aligned}&\textit{Somatotype attitudinal mean (SAM)}\\&= \frac{1.91 + 0.60 + 2.35 + 1.23 + 1.48 + 0.66 + 0.72}{7}\\&= 1.28\end{aligned}$$

Therefore, the SAM of the group is 1.28 (without there being any cut-off values to interpret this result).

7.7.4 Calculation of the Differences in the Somatotype Between One Group and Another Group

It allows establishing if a group is similar or different to another. For this, the dispersion distance of the mean somatotypes (DDMS) can be used, based on the X and Y coordinates, or the I index, based on the graphical representation of the somatotype in the somatochart.

1. Dispersion distance of the mean somatotypes (DDMS)

It serves to compare the mean somatotype of two groups based on their coordinates: Group 1 (X_{SM1}; Y_{SM1}) and Group 2 (X_{SM2}; Y_{SM2}).

$$\text{Dispersion distance of the mean somatotypes (DDMS)} = \sqrt{3*(X_{SM1} - X_{SM2})^2 + (Y_{SM1} - Y_{SM2})^2}$$

where:

- X_{SM1}: Value of the X coordinate calculated with the mean somatotype of the first group to compare.
- X_{SM2}: Value of the X coordinate calculated with the mean somatotype of the second group to compare.
- Y_{SM1}: Value of the Y coordinate calculated with the mean somatotype of the first group to compare.
- Y_{SM2}: Value of the Y coordinate calculated with the mean somatotype of the second group to compare.

It provides a number as the final value. If $SDD_{SM} > 2$, the differences are significant between the groups. But we are not going to know in which components the differences occur. Therefore, in case there are differences between groups, an analysis should be conducted to decide it is necessary to make any kind of adjustments to modify the mesomorphy or the endomorphy.

Next, an example is presented. In a club, there is a youth futsal team that competes in the honour division and another that competes in the regional division. The average somatotype of the first is 1.7 – 6.1 – 2.2 (0.48, 8.43) and the second's is 2.0 – 4.5 – 3.0 (1.00, 4.00).

The calculation of the DDMS to find if there are significant differences between both teams would be:

$$\begin{aligned}
&\text{Dispersion distance of the mean somatotypes (DDMS)}\\
&= \sqrt{3x(1.00 - 0.48)^2 + (4.00 - 8.43)^2}\\
&= \sqrt{3x(0.51)^2 + (-4.43)^2}\\
&= -\sqrt{3x0.26 + 19.61}\\
&= \sqrt{0.79 + 19.61}\\
&= \sqrt{20.4} = 4.52
\end{aligned}$$

Therefore, as the DDMS is 4.52 and is > 2, there are significant differences between the somatotypes of the two groups.

7.7.4.1 Index I

It serves to know if two or more groups are significantly different in a graphical way. For this, each group is represented with a somatopoint, whose coordinates are obtained with the application of the formulas X, Y of the somatotype obtained when calculating the mean somatotype (MS) of the group. From that point, a circle is drawn whose radius has the same length as the magnitude of the somatotype dispersion mean (SDM). In this way, in homogeneous groups, the radius will be smaller than in more heterogeneous groups. For the interpretation of Index I, it must be taken into account that if there is a common area between the two radii, there are no significant differences between the two groups. However, if there is no contact area between the circles, it is because the somatotype of both groups is significantly different.

Below is an example of how to calculate Index I with the previous data (the club that has a team in the honour division [1.7 – 6.1 – 2.2 (0.5, 8.3)] and another in regional [2.0 – 4.5 – 3.0 (1.0, 4.0)]).

The first thing is to represent the somatopoint of the average somatotype of each group on the somatochart. It can be found in Fig. 7.3.

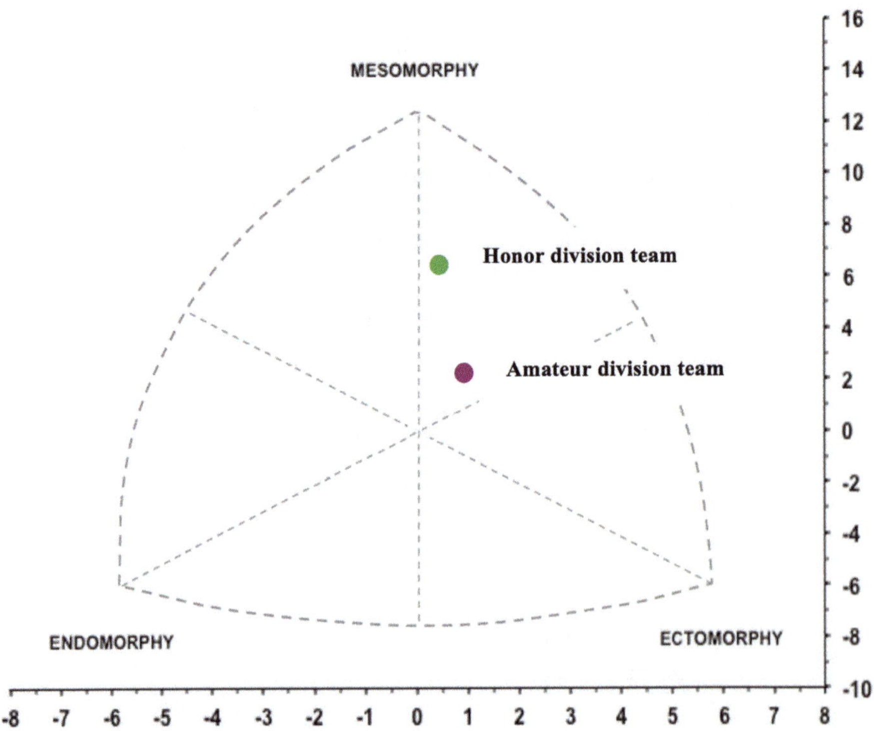

Fig. 7.3 Vertices of the somatochart and somatopoints

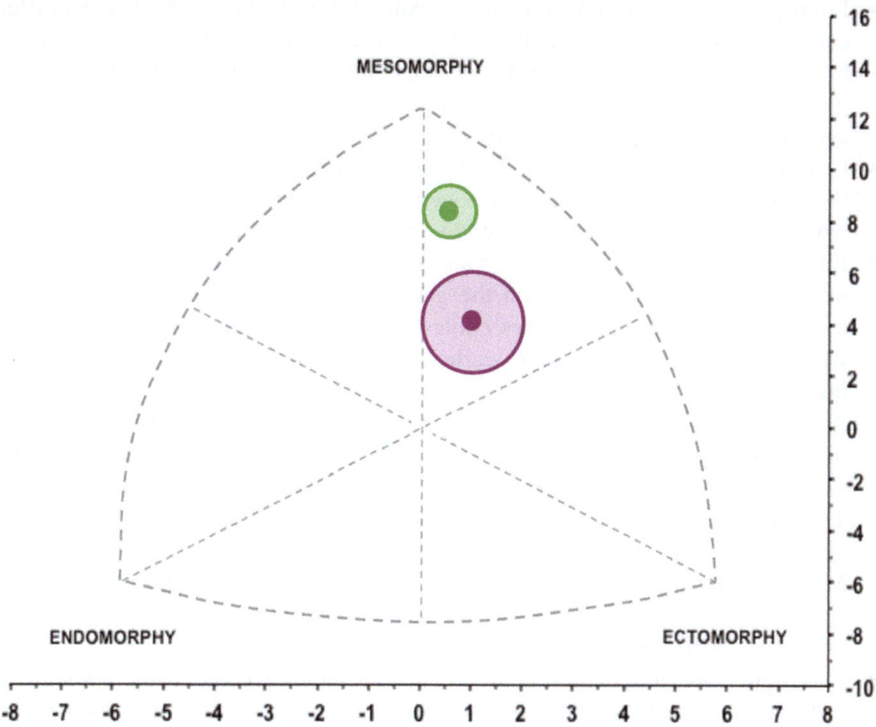

Fig. 7.4 Representation of the I-index of two groups on the somatochart

The next thing is to calculate the SDM of each group. Let's suppose that for the honour division group it is 0.5, and for the regional group it is 1. This is the radius of the circle that surrounds each somatopoint. This is shown in Fig. 7.4.

As the circles do not have a common area, it can be concluded that the groups are significantly different.

7.8 Aspects to Consider in the Application and Interpretation of the Somatotype

- With growth, changes occur in the somatotype as a result of biological maturation. Thus, the greatest changes occur from 6 to 12 years old, but during puberty, the somatotype continues to change.
- The changes that occur in adulthood are not strongly related to biological issues in general, but to factors of environmental origin, although it must be taken into account that both the ageing process and menopause result in specific changes in the somatotype during this stage. Thus, with ageing and menopause, endomorphy increases with age and ectomorphy slightly decreases.

- From puberty, a phenomenon called sexual dimorphism begins, that is, different morphological variations for each sex, which means that the morphotype of boys and girls is different in terms of shape, fat accumulation, and muscle development. Due to the above, starting in puberty, men will have less endomorphy and more mesomorphy than women.
- Ectomorphic children mature later and mesomorphs mature earlier. This is because the most determinant hormone in the maturation of boys is testosterone, which increases muscle mass, thereby explaining these differences.
- Endomorphic girls mature earlier and ectomorphic ones later. This is because maturation in girls depends on the generation of oestrogens, with this being a steroid hormone that requires cholesterol for its production, which explains why endomorphic girls mature earlier, while ectomorphic ones present a late maturation.
- Athletic performance benefits from a greater mesomorphy. Even at early ages, in certain sports such as contact sports, a greater endomorphy could also provide a competitive advantage for some aspects related to athletic performance. Therefore, early maturers, who present greater muscular development and, occasionally, fat, have a competitive advantage.
- Mesomorphy in athletes is greater than in inactive subjects, while endomorphy tends to be lower than in inactive subjects. In addition, an increase in training intensity corresponds with an increase in mesomorphy.
- The higher the athletic level, the greater the homogeneity of the somatotype of the groups, and therefore, the lower the dispersion of the somatotype of the athletes in the variables most related to athletic performance.
- The homogeneity of the somatotype is greater in individual sports than in team sports, because in team sports there are different positions and roles within the team. However, in tennis and cycling, despite being individual sports, there is great heterogeneity. The explanation in tennis is due to there being three competition surfaces, so the tennis players who perform on the same surface present great homogeneity, and similarly, in cycling, the athletes who are sprinters, climbers, or long-distance riders present characteristics similar to other cyclists who perform the same function.
- There are typical somatotypes for the practice of each sport. Thus, athletes in contact sports, combat, and in those where body mass is moved, are characterised by having a large mesomorphic component; and athletes with a high volume of aerobic work have a large ectomorphic component. In addition, there is specialised scientific literature on numerous sports modalities that enables us to find what we want an athlete who practices a certain modality to achieve in terms of values of endomorphy, mesomorphy and ectomorphy.

7.9 Questionnaire

1. Regarding the somatotype, indicate the false statement:
   (a) It is a method of quantifying the current shape and composition of the human body.
   (b) The somatotype is phenotypic, so environmental conditions and lifestyle habits cannot change it.
   (c) The somatotype cannot have negative values.
   (d) The somatotype provides a quantitative summary of the physique as a unified whole.
2. Indicate the true option regarding the components of the somatotype:
   (a) Endomorphy refers to relative adiposity.
   (b) Ectomorphy refers to relative linearity.
   (c) Mesomorphy refers to relative robustness.
   (d) All of the above are true.
3. Regarding the models used for the calculation of the somatotype:
   (a) The most currently used is the photoscopic method.
   (b) For the calculation with the anthropometric method, all the measurements of the complete ISAK profile are necessary.
   (c) The calculation of the somatotype using anthropometric measurements follows the method of Heath and Carter.
   (d) Although the anthropometric method is the most utilized, it is not the most useful because it provides little information.
4. Which of the following measurements is not used in the calculation of endomorphy?
   (a) Body mass.
   (b) Stretch stature.
   (c) Triceps skinfold.
   (d) Supraspinal skinfold.
5. Indicate the false one. the formulas used to calculate the corrected girths used in the mesomorphic component of the somatotype present handicaps because:
   (a) It uses the arm flexed and tensed girth and the triceps skinfold to correct it.
   (b) It does not multiply the skinfold by π to correct the girth.
   (c) There are no errors in the corrected girths of the somatotype.
   (d) The choice of variables in the correction of the calf girth is correct.
6. Regarding the results in the calculation of the somatotype, indicate the false one:
   (a) The resulting values cannot be negative.
   (b) It is unusual to find values less than 1 in endomorphy and mesomorphy.
   (c) If endomorphy and mesomorphy are high, ectomorphy will also be high.
   (d) Certain classifications of the somatotype are not biologically possible (2-2-2 or 7-8-7).
7. The graphical representation of the somatotype is the somatochart. indicate the true answer:

(a) The somatochart represents the three values that make up the somatotype separately.
(b) A subject with a somatotype 4-5-2 will be represented on the somatochart with the coordinates X = – 2, Y = 4.
(c) The somatotype cannot be represented in a two-dimensional graph because it has three dimensions.
(d) The X and Y axes of the somatochart are proportional.

8. Regarding the classification of the somatotype:
   (a) In Spanish there is some discrepancy regarding the exact translation of the terms used to classify the somatotype.
   (b) A somatotype represented numerically as 2-6-2, could be considered "balanced mesomorph".
   (c) When there is no predominant component, the somatotype is classified as *central*.
   (d) All are true.
9. Regarding the similarity or differentiation of the athlete compared to a group:
   (a) The somatotype dispersion distance (SDD) determines in which component of the somatotype a subject differs from the reference group.
   (b) The somatotype morphogenic distance (SAD) allows comparing the components of an individual's somatotype to a group.
   (c) It is not possible to compare the somatotype of different athletes because it changes.
   (d) All are false.
10. Regarding the aspects to consider about the somatotype:
   (a) The greatest changes occur in adulthood.
   (b) Ectomorphy increases with age, while endomorphy decreases.
   (c) High mesomorphy and moderate endomorphy are related to poorer motor performance in children.
   (d) In individual sports, with few exceptions, a greater homogeneity can be observed in the somatotype of high-level athletes.

Answers:
1.b 2.d 3.c 4.a 5.c 6.c 7.b 8.d 9.b 10.d

Bibliography

Carter, J. E. L., & Heath, B. H. (1990). *Somatotyping: Development and application.* Cambridge University Press.

Esparza-Ros, F. (1993). *Manual of Kinanthropometry.* FEMEDE.

Esparza-Ros, F., Vaquero-Cristóbal, R., & Marfell-Jones, M. (2019). *International protocol for anthropometric assessment.* International Society for the Advancement of Kinanthropometry.

Norton, K., & Olds, K. (1996). *Anthropometrica: A textbook of body measurement for sports and health courses.* UNSW Press.

Applying Anthropometry in Sport: From Talent Identification to Elite Sport

8

Abstract

Predicting sports performance requires a multifactorial approach. However, anthropometry has emerged as a key tool for assessing and predicting performance in various sports disciplines, allowing for talent identification and training optimisation. This chapter delves into the relationship between sports performance and body composition, especially referring to the fat and muscular component, or other anthropometric variables such as stretch stature, body mass, relative sitting height, relative length of the upper limb, brachial index, and acromial-iliac index. In addition, anthropometry is a key resource to consider in the process of detection and monitoring of sports talents. This chapter explains the need to approach the identification of sports talents from the perspective of anthropometric variables, with the consideration of biological maturation due to its influence on performance at growth ages being crucial. This chapter delves into the various methods to assess biological maturation.

Keywords

Sports performance • Anthropometry • Body composition • Maturation • Talent detection • Sports talent monitoring • Early maturer • Late maturer • On time maturer

8.1 Anthropometry and Sports Performance

Some authors define sports performance in competition as the athlete's ability to provide the appropriate response at each moment according to the specific demands of the sport they practice. Sports performance has always been one of the central concerns of sports professionals from different fields. Taking this definition into account, what makes an athlete become successful? The answer is not simple, as success is multifactorial. It has been observed that psychology, biomechanics,

© The Author(s), under exclusive license to Springer Nature Switzerland AG 2025

F. Esparza-Ros and R. Vaquero-Cristóbal, *Anthropometry*,
https://doi.org/10.1007/978-3-031-77535-2_8

technique, tactics, genetics, training, nutrition, rest, socioeconomic position, leisure activities, among other aspects, can affect sports performance.

Therefore, different tests have been designed to evaluate these variables in order to analyse the change of these aspects throughout the athlete's life, to be able to predict sports performance at different competitive levels, as well as apply the knowledge obtained in the design of detection, identification, and monitoring programmes for sports talents. This is why in recent years different variables have been used to discover the state of the athlete, such as the monitoring of physiological variables specific to each sports discipline, evaluations of psychological aspects, scales of perceived effort, nutritional assessment scales, technical and biomechanical assessment scales, different questionnaires and methodologies to carry out an evaluation of decision-making and tactical executions of individuals, or assessments of the general or specific physical condition of the sport. It should be noted that anthropometry has traditionally been found among the wide variety of existing tools for the assessment and characterisation of the requirements necessary for the optimal performance of an athlete.

Anthropometry is a useful tool in the study of the characteristics of successful athletes, as it allows finding and identifying the variables related to body shape and body composition that can be more determinant in the performance of the different sports disciplines. Among the variables that have been observed to have more influence on sports performance, we find.

8.1.1 Skinfolds and General Adiposity

In sports where active body mass movements are required, such as jumps, runs or sprints, a higher fat mass content is related to poorer performance, as it implies an increase in the athlete's body mass based on a tissue that does not directly contribute to the production of the necessary strength and power for these movements. Therefore, in general terms, a lower skinfold sum, a lower skinfold profile, and a lower adiposity, have been related to higher sports performance in different disciplines. This is true in most sports, but it has been especially observed that there is a great homogeneity of this statement in endurance sports, understanding these as aerobic effort sports, such as triathlon, cycling, swimming or medium and long distance races, and also team sports with few interruptions, such as football. This is because the most determining physical capacity in these disciplines is aerobic endurance, so the metabolic capacity can be limited by the accumulation of fat mass.

On the other hand, athletic modalities of jumps and sprints are explosive, short-duration sports, where the sports result of elite athletes is determined by small differences. Due to these specific characteristics, among the athletes who achieve high performance in these disciplines, a great homogeneity can be observed in the variables related to adiposity, such as fat mass and percentages, skinfold sums or the endomorphic component of the somatotype, variables in which they usually present relatively low values.

Regarding aesthetic sports, a great homogeneity can also be found in terms of variables related to adiposity. In this case, the reason is that the assessment of the athlete is not only based on objective performance parameters, but the assessment depends on subjective aspects, in which the body shape of the participants has a great influence. In these types of aesthetic modalities, such as synchronised swimming or rhythmic gymnastics, athletes can be found who present very low fat mass, and skinfold sums, due to the high volume of training required and the homogeneity of the body shape expected in competition, which can even increase the risk of eating disorders in athletes of these disciplines.

Finally, there are sports in which having a lower fat mass is a competitive advantage, although such homogeneity among athletes is no longer found, which means that this characteristic decreases in importance in order to reach the maximum performance of these sports. This can be observed in team sports with quick and discontinuous efforts and all the sports in which the rules allow numerous changes during the course of the competition, such as handball, indoor football, water polo, volleyball or basketball. These sports no longer depend as much on aerobic metabolic routes, but on anaerobic ones. And while it is true that excessive adiposity continues to be a competitive burden, in these sports, a greater heterogeneity can be found, as there is a high specificity in the functions that each athlete has to perform according to their position on the field, finding that athletes who have to maintain the position through body-to-body actions against an opponent, may see their performance benefited with a slightly higher fat mass. In addition, if an athlete is not in their optimal form, they can be substituted, which reduces the impact of this situation on collective performance.

In the case of combat sports, there is also a high heterogeneity, as in these sports, competition is based on body mass categories. A common practice in this type of sport is for the athlete to adjust their body mass to be included in a certain category in a quick way, in the last days before the competition. The purpose of this adjustment is to compete in a category that is lower than their real body mass, to try to gain a competitive advantage. Some studies have shown that most of the athletes who win combat sports competitions are very close to the maximum body mass allowed in the category. To be able to adjust to this body mass, which is usually lower than that of the athlete, a very severe food restriction is often carried out in the last few days prior to the competition, as well as high-intensity training aimed at promoting caloric expenditure and even dehydration. As it is not carried out in a sustained or orderly manner, the result is that they present a very heterogeneous fat profile, as it is more relevant to arrive within the body mass limit of the category than the fat mass of the athlete.

8.1.2 Corrected Girths, Transverse Muscle Areas and Percentage of Muscle Mass

In sports, there are a high number of actions that depend on the athlete's ability to generate strength and power. These abilities depend to some extent on neural and coordinative factors, but are largely related to the amount of muscle mass. This is why, in most sports, higher values in the corrected girths, the transverse muscle areas, and in the percentage of muscle mass, represent a competitive advantage. The greatest homogeneity with respect to the values presented in these variables is found in all the sports that depend, in terms of physical abilities, almost exclusively on strength and muscle power, such as combat sports and weightlifting. In these sports, very similar profiles can be found, characterised by very high muscle percentages, and the non-existence of another morphotype at the elite level, as it is not possible to perform well in these sports with moderate or low muscle percentages.

There is also homogeneity in this pattern in sports that depend on speed and agility, as they are also manifestations of strength and muscle power. Muscle development provides a competitive advantage in speed and agility sports, as the increase in contractile tissue allows technical actions to be executed at a higher speed. There is a high of homogeneity in terms of the high muscle percentage in team sports, in the athletics modalities that depend on jumping and speed, and in swimming.

In endurance sports, muscle mass is not the most determining factor. The most determining factor is the low fat mass. This means that in these sports, there is a heterogeneous profile with respect to muscle mass. Thus, there are athletes within these modalities who manage to perform with very high muscle percentages, but there are also other athletes who manage to perform with more moderate muscle percentages. This is because having an excess of muscle percentage in these types of sports can be a competitive burden, as a high muscle mass in aerobic sports can worsen the required energy efficiency, so athletes with different characteristics can perform in the same manner.

8.1.3 Individual Anthropometric Variables

Once the plastic components of body composition (muscle and fat mass) have been analysed, some anthropometric variables that have also been strongly related to sports performance will be discussed. When discussing the characterisation of the anthropometric requirements of the different sports disciplines, it should be taken into account that the greater the homogeneity shown by elite athletes in a certain anthropometric variable, the greater influence can be attributed to it in sports success, and therefore, the absence of this characteristic will greatly hinder the individual's ability to perform at the highest level in that discipline.

8.1.3.1 Stretch Stature

The stretch stature variable is strongly influenced by genetics (Factor 0.85, i.e., 85% conditioned by exclusively genetic factors). In addition, high-performance athletes usually have a greater stretch stature than the general population, and stretch stature presents a competitive advantage in most sports. All of this has led to attempts to use stretch stature in the detection of sports talents, through the use of different equations to try to predict the stretch stature that young athletes can reach in their adult stage.

Athletes with a greater stretch stature have a competitive advantage in sports such as swimming; tennis, especially on grass; net sports such as volleyball; or sports where the goal is high, as is the case with basketball. There have also been sports where a greater stretch stature, having proportionally a larger trunk, can provide a competitive advantage when performing a certain mechanical movement, as is the case with rowing. On the contrary, there are other sports in which a shorter stretch stature provides a competitive advantage, such as aesthetic sports, as they require great stability, and a shorter stretch stature means having the centre of gravity closer to the ground, making the athletes more stable. Similarly, in sports such as climbing, a shorter stretch stature can enhance performance, as when moving along a wall all limbs are closer to each other, so that more force can be applied from the trunk and with a more efficient force transmission.

8.1.3.2 Body Mass

Body mass, especially when due to an increase in muscle mass, provides a competitive advantage in all contact sports, throwing, sports where you have to lift a certain body mass, or in sports where you have to exert force. However, it is also true that in endurance and aesthetic sports, which are strongly associated to fat mass, a higher performance often depends on having a low body mass.

8.1.3.3 Relative Sitting Height

The relative sitting height refers to the relationship between sitting height and stretch stature, so that a person with a higher relative sitting height has a proportionally higher sitting height measurement (proportionally longer trunk and proportionally shorter legs) than another individual with a lower relative sitting height (proportionally shorter trunk and proportionally longer legs). A higher relative sitting height provides a competitive advantage in combat sports and in sports where the athlete has to lift a certain load, such as weightlifting. This is due to a biomechanical fact, as the shorter the fulcrum (trunk) is in relation to the load that needs to be overcome, and the closer the centre of gravity is to the ground (fulcrum), the more efficient the application of forces will be. On the contrary, a low relative sitting height provides a competitive advantage in all sports that depend on jumps, races, or leg traction.

8.1.3.4 Relative Length of the Upper Limb

This measurement relates the length of the upper limb (arm + forearm + hand), and stretch stature. It has been found that, in sports such as swimming, synchronised diving, water polo, rowing or boxing, that is, in most sports where the movement starts from the upper limb, a greater relative length of the upper limb is a competitive advantage. On the contrary, in sports where large loads need to be moved, efficiency improves if these are as close as possible to the trunk. Therefore, having a proportionally shorter upper limb is a competitive advantage, as it allows moving loads close to the base of support and the trunk, where the stabilising muscles and the muscles that exert a greater force in the movement when exerting maximum force are located. This is the case, for example, with weightlifting.

8.1.3.5 Brachial Index

The brachial index is the relationship between the length of the forearm and the arm. A higher brachial index indicates that the forearm is proportionally larger than the arm. Based on this index, athletes of modalities in which the forearm is used as a support point and the elbow as the axis of movement benefit from a higher index, as is the case with swimming in freestyle style, where the movement starts from the shoulder and the entire arm is used, but the lever is applied from the elbow joint, using the hand and forearm to push the water, or in slalom canoeing, where the movements to adjust the canoe start from the elbow. In this type of sports, it is of interest that the transmission of forces is as efficient as possible, so the shorter the arm the better. On the contrary, a low brachial index, that is, a forearm proportionally shorter than the upper arm, will provide an advantage in most combat sports, as a greater transmission of forces from the shoulder is achieved, or in sports where high loads need to be moved, as is the case with weightlifting, by preventing the load from moving away from the trunk in different planes.

8.1.3.6 Acromial-Iliac Index

The acromial-iliac index is the relationship between the biiliocristal breadth (hip width) and the biacromial breadth (shoulder width). This difference in the proportionality of the two breadths between sports disciplines may be related to the "library effect". This theory, developed by Francis Holway, argues that due to the structural function of the bone system, if the athlete's bone structure is larger, it can contain more mass composed of plastic tissues, whether muscle or fat mass, while if the structure is smaller, the mass it can contain will be more limited. Thus, according to the "library effect" theory, the biiliocristal breadth better predicts the individual's body mass than stretch stature, since there is a greater limitation in terms of the range of body mass that an individual can have depending on the proportionality of their trunk than by their stretch stature. This is because the trunk is where most of an individual's body mass is found, as it contains the organs and a large concentration of the blood and visceral fat mass, and there is also a large amount of muscle mass and visceral fat.

According to this theory, in strength sports, a large structure will be more beneficial, allowing for a greater muscle mass to be contained. On the other hand, in endurance sports a proportionally large trunk is not beneficial, as excessive body mass in an endurance sport leads to a competitive disadvantage. Thus, in this type of sports, a lower acromial-iliac index is of interest, as it allows for a smaller mass to be contained. Therefore, it has been found that in endurance sports, a lower acromial-iliac index may be related to better performance, with indices below 1.4 being common in these athletes. That is, the biacromial breadth is proportionally smaller as compared to the biiliocristal breadth. On the other hand, in sports where strength is paramount, it is common to find acromio-iliac indices greater than 1.46, that is, the biacromial breadth is proportionally larger as compared to the biiliocristal breadth.

8.2 Anthropometry and Sport in the Training Age

With respect to sport in the training age, two phenomena occur; the process of talent detection in sports and the process of identification and monitoring of talents. The detection of sports talents consists of selecting young athletes with good prospects for achieving high performance in their discipline. This process is commonly used by sports clubs with large financial budgets and a large number of participants, who can afford not to select those individuals who do not show the necessary characteristics to reach the elite at the time of selection, with the clearest example being football.

Regarding the identification and monitoring of sports talents, it has been defined as the monitoring of young athletes to try to provide training opportunities and motor development to those who are most likely to reach the elite, without this meaning neglecting the rest of the subjects. This process is more commonly used in sports modalities with a smaller budget that also tend to have fewer participants; or for the more modest teams of the most popular sports.

For decades, there has been a great interest in identifying, from a young age, which athletes will have more chances of performing well in a certain sport. This is due, in the first place, to the fact that being able to prematurely determine which athletes are most likely to perform well in a certain sport allows for early specialisation of the skills that will most determine sports performance in later stages, both technically and tactically, and of those physical abilities that will most influence sports performance, in such a way that a young athlete can be obtained, who will already have all the abilities when they reach their teenage stage, to promote the sports performance of that sport. These types of models also offer the possibility of incorporating young players into top-level teams. The fact of having pre-selected athletes around the start of adolescence makes so that the athlete can be integrated into the elite team, once they have passed their peak growth age and morphological adaptations begin to occur, such as an increase in muscle and bone mass, and if training has been carried out in the technical-tactical abilities necessary to achieve good performance. On the other hand, these types of early talent identification programmes bring some economic stability to the clubs that implement them, as the resources that are allocated to the development of a training plan for athletes in the growth stage bring with them a decrease in spending on the incorporation of athletes from outside the club.

However, there are also detractors of this methodology of identification and early specialisation of sports talents. Most of the detractors base their arguments on an approach oriented towards sports pedagogy. What they promote is that, in the case of early specialisation, if that athlete does not manage to achieve the expected performance in that sport, they will abandon sports practice or be discarded in the selection process, while if the athlete at an early age acquires a sufficient motor background to be able to practice a great diversity of sports activities, they will have more opportunities for practice and more enriching experiences. Currently, the differences between the interests of sports clubs seeking performance and the pedagogical approach to sports practice is one of the most controversial issues around the identification of sports talents.

Traditionally, these early talent identification programmes in sports have been based on the characterisation of the requirements in terms of physical abilities and anthropometric variables of adult athletes, to later try to identify young athletes with similar characteristics. However, it is worth noting that adolescent athletes who usually stand out in identification programmes have a common characteristic, as they present a more advanced maturation process than their peers. The influence of the maturation process on anthropometric variables and physical condition makes it difficult to know how to make assessments to be able to identify sports talent with certain guarantees, and that is why in recent years, many studies have been carried out to try to predict which variable should be considered when identifying sports talents. It has been shown that it is necessary to carry out a technical-tactical analysis to observe how the athlete behaves, including both technical aspects and problem-solving situations, to analyse the implementation of tactical aspects. Also, it has been observed that physical performance must also be evaluated, as it affects sports performance. In most sports, there are certain physical abilities that will determine performance in that sport. Finally, it has been observed that those anthropometric variables with the greatest genetic influence have to be evaluated in order to correctly identify sports talents. Therefore, the three groups of variables that traditionally form part of sports identification models are technical-tactical qualities, physical performance, and anthropometric variables. But these are not the only ones, as there are other factors that could help identify sports talents, such as psychological characteristics, or sociodemographic factors, which include the level of education of the parents, the level of education of the athletes, the capacity for effort, or the economic status.

The aforementioned factors are related to the performance of athletes in training, but one must also consider that the current performance of a growing athlete does not necessarily have to be related to their future performance; nor do the anthropometric characteristics of the athlete in training largely predict the anthropometric characteristics of the athlete in the future. In this sense, one of the main problems is that until a few years ago, the influence of biological maturation on the variables that were traditionally included in sports talent identification programmes had not been taken into account. This has caused athletes who matured earlier to have a higher probability of being selected. That is why it is necessary to monitor athletes to find what their maturation status is, what their current performance is, and based on their maturation status, what their future performance could be.

8.2.1 Biological Maturation

Biological maturation is understood, in relation to human growth, as the set of physical, physiological, and psychological changes that take place from birth until reaching adult maturation development. These changes become especially relevant around puberty, due to the speed at which they occur.

The set of processes that shape biological maturation is not uniform, with differences observed in the rate of maturation between sexes and inter-individual differences. In fact, it is a process that can be influenced by exogenous factors, such as the fat mass present before puberty. Thus, it has been observed that a greater accumulation of fat mass favours the early onset of maturation processes, especially in women. For physical activity, it has been observed that subjects who practice sports disciplines whose peak performance occurs at early ages and who have large volumes and intensities of training, such as sports and rhythmic gymnastics, may have their maturation process delayed, or that a low caloric availability, either due to nutritional deficit or training load, could also delay the onset of pubertal maturation.

In different studies, it has been shown that men usually have the onset of puberty between the ages of 12 and 15.8, while in the case of women, the onset of puberty usually appears between the ages of 9.3 and 15. Until this maturation occurs, the physical characteristics of boys and girls are very similar, and it is from this point on that large changes begin to occur and sexual dimorphism is more observable, so boys and girls begin to have large differences in their shape and body composition.

In relation to biological maturation, two concepts stand out, which are chronological age and biological age:

- Chronological age, known simply as "age", refers to the time elapsed from the subject's birth to a certain moment in their life. It is important that during the different stages of growth, the chronological age be calculated in a decimal way, as at a maturation level, there can be many differences between an child who is 12 years old, but is going to turn 13 in a month (12.9 years), than an child who is 12 years old and just turned that age a month ago (12.1 years).
- Biological age is the age in relation to some maturation indicator that a certain individual presents. Biological age does not have to coincide with chronological age, giving rise to the concept "maturation lag", understood as the difference between chronological age and biological age (in years).

  One of the indicators of biological maturation most used in young athletes is the age at which the peak height velocity (APHV) occurs, due to its relationship with numerous hormonal and physical changes. The peak height velocity is the age at which an individual is going to show the moment of maximum growth speed in stretch stature and body mass. The result of the APHV calculation is expressed in years. If the resulting value of the APHV calculation is negative, it means that the individual lacks those specific years to reach the moment of maximum growth, whereas, if the value is positive, it means that the individual

Table 8.1 Example of calculation of chronological age, maturational lag and effects of age at peak height velocity (APHV)

	Subject 1	Subject 2	Subject 3
Chronological age	13 years-old	13 years-old	13 years-old
APHV	12 years	13 years	15.5 years
Maturational lag	+ 1	0	− 2.5

APHV: age at peak height velocity

passed that moment those years ago. For example, three individuals of the same chronological age, 13 years, can have three different APHVs (Table 8.1).

With the APHV value, we can determine whether an individual is a normal maturer, early mature, or late maturer:

- Early maturer: their peak growth occurs before 13.4 years for boys and before 11.4 years for girls.
- Normal maturer: their peak growth occurs between 13.4 and 14.4 years for boys and between 11.4 and 12.2 years for girls.
- Late maturer: the peak growth occurs after 14.4 years for boys and after 12.2 years for girls.

The ages at which this APHV can be calculated are those between 12 and 15.8 for boys, and from 9.3 to 15 years for girls. Outside these ranges, the calculation of maturation would be meaningless, as most methods used for its calculation lose sensitivity in terms of individual differences once the majority of changes have already occurred.

8.2.1.1 Methods of Assessing Biological Maturation

There are different methods for calculating the APHV depending on the indicator of biological maturation being studied.

Radiographic Methods: Based on the State of the Epiphyses

The *gold standard* for estimating the APHV is the hand and wrist radiograph, with which the skeletal age is calculated. Through this test, the state of the epiphyses of the ulna and radius and the state of development and calcification of the wrist bones are observed. If the person has not reached the peak of growth, the epiphyses will be less calcified. Thus, this method is based on the fact that in young people the epiphyses are still connective tissue, while in those people who have passed that moment of maximum growth it is already bone tissue.

Marshall-Tanner Method: Based on the Development of the Sexual Characteristics

This method is based on comparing the development of the individual's sexual characteristics with a scale divided into five stages. A scale has been developed for boys and another for girls. This method has some limitations in its application by non-medical personnel. Originally, it was a method developed for use in clinical practice by medical personnel, so outside the clinical setting it is not considered ethical to use it through direct observation. This leaves self-completion by the subject as the only method of use, which can lead to errors in identifying the stage at which their development of sexual characteristics is found. On the other hand, another limitation is the narrow time frame in which it can be used, as before the onset of the development of sexual characteristics it cannot be used, nor once full development has been reached.

Somatic Maturation: Based on Anthropometric Measures

This method is based on the relationship and proportionality between different anthropometric measurements to estimate the APHV. In this case, to estimate it, a formula developed by Mirwald et al. (2002) is applied, in which the length of the lower limb (stretch stature – sitting height), age, sex, and body mass, can be used to estimate the APHV. This is highly interesting, as it is a very simple formula, being based on anthropometric measurements. It provides very interesting information about the rate of maturation of an individual, and it even allows them to be classified as early, on time, or late maturer as compared to the group.

$$\begin{aligned}\text{Boys} = {} & -9.236 + 0.0002708 * (\text{Lower limb length (cm)} * \text{sitting height (cm)}) \\ & - 0.001663 * (\text{decimal age} * \text{lower limb length (cm)}) \\ & + 0.007216 * ((\text{decimal age} * \text{sitting height (cm)}) \\ & + 0.02292 * (\text{body mass (kg)}/\text{stretch stature (cm)})\end{aligned}$$

$$\begin{aligned}\text{Girls} = {} & -9.376 + 0.0001882 * (\text{lower limb length (cm)} * \text{sitting height (cm)}) \\ & + 0.0022 * (\text{decimal age} * \text{lower limb length (cm)}) \\ & + 0.005841 * (\text{decimal age} * \text{sitting height (cm)}) \\ & - 0.002658 * (\text{age} * \text{body mass (kg)}) \\ & + 0.07693 * (\text{body mass (kg)}/\text{stretch stature(cm)})\end{aligned}$$

where:

- Lower limb length (cm): Stretch stature (cm) – Sitting height (cm).

Dental Maturation: Based on the Development of the Teeth

This method is based on dental radiography to estimate the biological age from the development of the teeth. It has a wide range of applicability from birth to adult development, and a high validity and reliability. However, it is not without limitations, as it requires highly specialised personnel for its implementation, as well as specific facilities and equipment that is not easily accessible, which does not allow its adaptation to field measurements, so it is rarely used in field work.

8.2.1.2 Biological Maturation, Anthropometry and Sports Performance

The importance of predicting APHV occurs is the great increase in muscle mass and bone mass in both sexes at this time and from that point on, mainly due to the fact that in both boys and girls, the testosterone levels increase, with these levels being higher in boys. On the other hand, there is a progressive increase of the fat mass during the maturation stage, mainly in the girl population. Indeed, it has been observed that early maturing women have a greater fat mass as compared to their chronological age peers who mature later. It should not be forgotten that oestrogens are some of the main hormones responsible for maturation in the case of girls, and these are steroid hormones, which require a lipid component for their composition. On the contrary, in the case of boys, the maintenance of fat mass is observed during the maturation stage.

In the case of stretch stature, its development largely depends on the growth hormone and its levels greatly increase around the APHV, so this would be another aspect to consider in terms of the detection of sporting talents. It should also be considered that heights, body masses, sitting heights, and other bone and structural variables that depend on the concentrations of growth hormone in young athletes who are at different stages of biological maturation, should not be compared. Similarly, the influence of maturation on physical abilities related to strength and its manifestation, and sports in which a greater body mass and a greater stretch stature are a competitive advantage, should be taken into account.

Therefore, an athlete who reaches the peak of growth before others of his/her same chronological age, and who, therefore, develops a greater muscle mass, bone mass, stretch stature and in some cases even fat mass, is likely to have a competitive advantage until the maturation rates are equalised with the rest of the group, as these variables influence physical condition and therefore, influence the athletic performance of the subject in most sports.

In fact, recent research has shown that pubertals who were early maturers jumped higher, threw further, had more strength in the lower limb and in the upper limb, were able to have a greater speed and had a greater agility. Therefore, in all sports in which having greater strength, being faster or having greater agility is a competitive advantage, early maturers will have a competitive advantage until the rest of the pubertals do not reach that moment of maturation. However, it seems that there are no differences according to the rate of maturation in aerobic endurance or flexibility.

The fact that maturation not only generates adaptations in anthropometric variables, but these adaptations are directly manifested in physical abilities that have to do with the production of power and strength, may be due to the fact that before the APHV occurs, the lack of availability of testosterone means that the adaptations that occur with training are not at a morphological level, but are at a neural and coordinative level. After the APHV, adaptations occur in two ways; at the neural level, and through morphological adaptations. Thus, early maturers who reach the APHV before their peers and who start to generate testosterone have two different types of adaptations to the same stimulus than the pubertal who has yet mature, and this gives them a competitive advantage. On the other hand, endurance and flexibility are not strongly influenced by testosterone, and therefore, are not so affected by maturation, although they are strongly influenced by training adaptation.

Therefore, when detecting, identifying, and monitoring sporting talents, some considerations must be taken into account. If tests related to strength, speed, and agility are intended to be carried out, in the case that there are different ranges of maturation in the evaluated athletes, it will be necessary to take into account the modulating effect of maturation on the results obtained. However, in the case of those tests related to aerobic endurance and flexibility, comparisons can be made without much concern for maturation. Regarding anthropometric variables, in the case of boys, early maturers have a greater body mass, greater stretch stature, greater sitting height, greater body mass index, and greater muscle and bone development, but no differences are observed in fat mass. In the case of girls, the findings are similar, with differences also observed in fat content.

In conclusion, the processes of selection, detection and monitoring of sporting talents are complex and multifactorial. From the perspective of anthropometric variables, one should consider whether a young athlete who is an early mature, with characteristics that give him/her an advantage during the growth stage over his/her peers, will continue to stand out from the group once the maturation process is concluded. In sports, only immediate performance has mattered for many years, so changing this trend for the implementation of long-term monitoring and tracking of athletes is not an easy task. One should consider whether individuals who reach the elite of a particular sport have achieved sporting success because of natural selection, in which all athletes have been offered similar development, motor and competitive opportunities, and therefore, those who have reached the elite are have a more suitable biological, genetic, technical-tactical, sociodemographic, psychological, etc. predisposition to achieve the best sporting performance, or if, on the contrary, selection pressure was applied, where more development opportunities were provided to the individuals who stood out from the rest of the athletes at an early age, which usually coincides in most sports with early maturers, leaving aside those who did not show the necessary characteristics to succeed during the growth stage. In the second case, it should be taken into account that the differences in the characteristics that make these adolescents have a competitive advantage at that time, may be equalised in the future with the progress of the maturation process.

In relation to this, there is a problem in the organisation of grassroots sports, in that the competitions in these sports are grouped by chronological ages, generally every two natural years, in such a way that there are adolescents who have the same chronological age, but have completely different biological ages. Therefore, in the end, early maturers will have more motor opportunities due to selection pressure, so they will consequently have a greater motor background, a greater number of opportunities, and a greater probability of reaching professional or high performance levels of sport. On the other hand, the athlete who is a late maturer, as a result of the disadvantage during puberty, does not have enough motor opportunities to be able to fully develop, even if the biological conditions were eventually equalised.

However, success during puberty does not guarantee future success, with numerous studies having shown that athletes who manage to have greater successes at the elite level are those who were late maturers in their day. And this is because the late maturers, despite having a great disadvantage, managed to maintain the same level as their peers, and when conditions are equalised at the end of maturation, they are likely to have many more resources to perform in elite sport.

For all these arguments, it would be advisable to readjust the competitive categories at training ages, and the models of identification of sporting talents should be carried out that take into account the maturation status and its influence on specific and general performance in order to also offer opportunities to late maturers.

8.3 Questionnaire

1. Indicate the true statement:
   (a) Anthropometry is not used for the evaluation of elite athletes.
   (b) Anthropometry has not been used to characterise training athletes.
   (c) Anthropometry is one of the tools that has traditionally been used in the evaluation of elite and training athletes.
   (d) All are false.
2. As a general rule:
   (a) A greater fat mass is related to worse sports performance.
   (b) Fat mass is of little relevance in endurance sports.
   (c) Fat mass is of extreme relevance in team sports with unlimited changes.
   (d) Fat mass directly contributes to the production of strength.
3. Regarding corrected girths, muscular areas and muscle mass:
   (a) They are not highly relevant in most sports.
   (b) A very high percentage of muscle mass is associated with better performance in aesthetic sports.
   (c) Higher values in these variables are associated with a greater ability to produce strength and power.
   (d) In sports that depend on speed or agility, there can be heterogeneity in the values of these variables among different athletes.
4. Stretch stature is one of the anthropometric variables that have been shown to influence sports performance. Indicate the true one:
   (a) Stretch stature is greatly influenced by genetics.
   (b) High-performance athletes tend to be taller than the general population.
   (c) A short stretch stature can be a competitive advantage in certain sports.
   (d) All are true.

5. A higher relative sitting height can be an advantage in sports such as:
   (a) Volleyball.
   (b) Weightlifting.
   (c) High jump.
   (d) Sprint races (100 m, 200 m).
6. A greater relative length of the upper limb is related to:
   (a) Better performance in sports where the movement starts from the arms.
   (b) Better performance in sports where large load movements are performed.
   (c) Better performance in sports where jumps and races predominate.
   (d) There is no relationship between the relative length of the upper limb and sports performance.
7. The "library effect" in relation to anthropometry refers to:
   (a) The number of books on anthropometry and sports performance that exist.
   (b) The function of fat mass in certain sports disciplines.
   (c) The function of the bone structure in the accumulation of plastic tissues, whether muscle or fat mass.
   (d) None of the above.
8. Within the models of identification of sports talents:
   (a) Anthropometry has been used to characterise the requirements of sports disciplines in terms of the morphology of elite athletes.
   (b) The aim was to ensure that the young athletes selected had anthropometric characteristics similar to those of elite athletes.
   (c) Traditionally, no attention was paid to the influence of biological maturation on the anthropometric variables of young athletes.
   (d) All are true.
9. Among the methods of estimating biological maturation:
   (a) The method based on hand and wrist radiography is unreliable.
   (b) The APHV can be estimated using anthropometric variables and specific formulas for each sex.
   (c) Sexual maturation is the method whose age range in which it can be applied is wider.
   (d) Dental maturation is the method most used in fieldwork.
10. Early maturers, both boys and girls:
   (a) They usually present higher values in muscle and bone mass variables compared to late maturers.
   (b) They do not present competitive advantages during adolescence.
   (c) They tend to have fewer development opportunities when selection pressures are exerted.
   (d) They usually present a smaller stretch stature and body mass compared to late maturers.

Answers:
1.c 2.a 3.c 4.d 5.b 6.a 7.c 8.d 9.b 10.a

Bibliography

Albaladejo-Saura, M., Vaquero-Cristóbal, R., González-Gálvez, N., & Esparza-Ros, F. (2021). Relationship between biological maturation, physical fitness, and kinanthropometric variables of young athletes: A systematic review and meta-analysis. *International Journal of Environmental Research & Public Health, 18*(1), 328.

Albaladejo-Saura, M., Vaquero-Cristóbal, R., García-Roca, J. A., & Esparza-Ros, F. (2022a). Influence of biological maturation status on selected anthropometric and physical fitness variables in adolescent male volleyball players. *PeerJ, 10*, e13216.

Albaladejo-Saura, M., Vaquero-Cristóbal, R., García-Roca, J. A., & Esparza-Ros, F. (2022b). Influence of maturity status on kinanthropometric and physical fitness variables in adolescent female volleyball players. *Applied Sciences, 12*, 4400.

Albaladejo-Saura, M., Vaquero-Cristóbal, R., García-Roca, J. A., & Esparza-Ros, F. (2022c). The effect of age, biological maturation and birth quartile in the kinanthropometric and physical fitness differences between male and female adolescent volleyball players. *Children, 9*(1), 58.

Beunen, G. P., Malina, R. M., Lefevre, J., Claessens, A. L., Renson, R., Eynde, B. K., Vanreusel, B., & Simons, J. (1997). Skeletal maturation, somatic growth and physical fitness in girls 6–16 years of age. *International Journal of Sports Medicine, 18*(6), 413–419.

Cabañas, M. D., & Esparza, F. (2009). *Compendium of Kinanthropometry*. CTO Editorial.

Demirjian, A., & Goldstein, H. (1976). New systems for dental maturity based on seven and four teeth. *Annals of Human Biology, 3*(5), 411–421.

Katzmarzyk, P. T., Malina, R. M., & Beunen, G. P. (1997). The contribution of biological maturation to the strength and motor fitness of children. *Annals of Human Biology, 24*(6), 493–505.

Malina, R. M., & Bouchard, C. (1991). *Growth, maturation, and physical activity*. Human Kinetics Books.

Marshall, W. A., & Tanner, J. M. (1969). Variations in pattern of pubertal changes in girls. *Archives of Disease in Childhood, 44*(235), 291–303.

Marshall, W. A., & Tanner, J. M. (1970). Variations in the pattern of pubertal changes in boys. *Archives of Disease in Childhood, 45*(239), 13–23.

Mirwald, R. L., Baxter-Jones, A. D., Bailey, D. A., & Beunen, G. P. (2002). An assessment of maturity from anthropometric measurements. *Medicine & Sciences in Sports and Exercise, 34*(4), 689–694.

Applying Anthropometry in Health: Identification and Diagnosis of Diseases

9

Abstract

Anthropometry is crucial in the field of health due to its usefulness in the prevention and monitoring of chronic diseases and risk groups. This chapter carries out an analysis of the anthropometric variables most related to different pathologies, in order to identify risk factors and provide information about the health of the individual, underlining body mass, skinfolds, waist and hips girths, waist/hip, waist/ stretch stature and stretch stature/wrist girth ratios, the body mass index (BMI), adiposity, somatotype, and the conicity index. Finally, an analysis of the anthropometric variables most related to anorexia nervosa, diabetes, cardiovascular pathology, and obesity, is carried out.

Keywords

Health • Chronic diseases • Anthropometry • Obesity • Diabetes • Cardiovascular pathology • Conicity index • Body mass index • Waist/hip ratio

9.1 Applications of Anthropometry in the Field of Health

Anthropometry has a great importance in the field of health due to its proven usefulness in the prevention and monitoring of various pathologies. Among its main applications, we find:

- Identifying the anthropometric characteristics of people at risk of developing certain pathologies.
- Identifying the anthropometric characteristics of people who are suffering from certain pathologies.

© The Author(s), under exclusive license to Springer Nature Switzerland AG 2025

F. Esparza-Ros and R. Vaquero-Cristóbal, *Anthropometry*,
https://doi.org/10.1007/978-3-031-77535-2_9

- Delving into the mechanisms that underpin a certain pathology.
- Guiding health interventions.
- Monitoring the effects of interventions.

Therefore, two main utilities of anthropometry in the area of health are identified: the identification and prevention of risk groups (anorexia, obesity, diabetes, cardiovascular pathology or metabolic syndrome, among others), and the monitoring of the effects of a treatment carried out in populations with pathology.

9.2 Most Determining Anthropometric Measurements in the Field of Health

In the field of health, for prevention and the identification of risk groups, there are thirteen most commonly utilized anthropometric measurements, with one of these belonging to the complete profile, while the remaining ones to the ISAK restricted profile. The twelve measurements of the restricted profile are: body mass, stretch stature, eight skinfolds (triceps, subscapular, biceps, iliac crest, supraspinal, abdominal, thigh and calf), waist and hips girths; and one from the complete profile described by ISAK: the antero-posterior abdominal breadth. These are the most determinant in the identification of risk factors, and provide more information in relation to the health of the individual. It should be noted that, within this selection, the most used are body mass, stretch stature, the triceps, subscapular, supraspinal and abdominal skinfolds and the waist and hips girths.

More specifically, each of these measurements has specific characteristics in relation to the field of health, which are outlined below:

- Body mass: it is a routine measurement in any health-related anthropometric profile, as excessive body mass and its excessive variability are associated with different pathologies.

  Fluctuations in body mass with cyclical increases and decreases are related to greater glucose intolerance, insulin resistance, and increased blood pressure, while the reduction of body mass decreases the risk of longevity loss caused by type 2 diabetes, in hypertensive subjects this loss of body mass is related to the normalisation of blood pressure, and is also related to the increase in HDL and the decrease in LDL and triglycerides.
- Skinfolds: these can be used to locate the distribution of fat mass, differentiating two groups of adiposity distribution:
  - Gynoid distribution, characterised by an accumulation of fat mass in the buttocks and thighs, being typical in women.
  - Android distribution, characterised by an accumulation of fat mass in the abdominal region, being typical in men.

- Skinfolds located in the trunk (subscapular, iliac crest, supraspinal and abdominal) provide more information about an individual's health than peripheral skinfolds (biceps, triceps, thigh and leg). This is because the skinfolds located in the trunk have a positive correlation with high blood pressure, elevated triglycerides, high body mass index (BMI), angina pectoris and morbidity-mortality from cardiovascular diseases.
- It is worth noting that the ratio of subscapular/triceps skinfolds provides a representative value on the incidence of mortality in women, as the accumulation of fat mass in the triceps of women is usually quite high, so an index above 1, in which the subscapular skinfold is higher than the triceps, would indicate a large accumulation of fat mass in the trunk. This ratio has a direct relationship with ischemic heart disease and mortality from cardiovascular etiopathogenesis in women.
- Girths: one of the most utilized health indices is the waist/hip ratio, although very notable modifications of fat mass are required before this index changes in value.

  Both the waist and hips girths are indicators of adipose distribution, with the hips girth referring to peripheral adiposity, and the waist to visceral adiposity. Therefore, the waist/hip ratio correlates with the content of visceral fat mass in the body. An increase in the value of this index indicates an increase in visceral fat mass at the expense of superficial adiposity and, therefore, a higher cardiovascular risk.

  The reference health values established for this index are: in women below 0.85 (normality between 0.71 and 0.85) and in men below 0.90 (normality between 0.78 and 0.90), with values higher than those indicated related to an exponential increase in cardiovascular risk and arteriosclerotic pathologies.

  Another index of special relevance for calculating cardiovascular risk in adults between 25 and 60 years old is the waist-to-height ratio (waist girth/stretch stature) (WHtR). The probability of presenting cardiovascular risk factors increases from a value of 0.53 in men and 0.51 in women. In infants, the WHtR presents a good correlation with fat mass through the skinfolds, with values between 0.48 and 0.51 found in overweight children, and values above 0.51 in obese children; whereas in overweight girls, the value lies between 0.47–0.50, and in obese girls, it is above 0.50.

  Body build (stretch stature/wrist girth) determines the size of a person's body structure. The build will be small if the value is above 10.1 in men and 10.9 in women; medium if it is between 10.1–9.6 in men and 10.9–9.9 in women; and large if the value is below 9.6 in men and 9.9 in women.

9.3 Body Composition as a Health Indicator

The accumulation of excess adiposity leads to clinical obesity and is related to mortality in men and cardiovascular pathology in both men and women.

Table 9.1 Body mass index (BMI) classification

Under weight	< 18.4
Normal weight	18.5–24.9
Overweight	24.9–30.0
Obesity I	30.0–34.9
Obesity II	35.0–39.9
Obesity III	> 40.0

Since 1869, the BMI, which relates body mass and stretch stature: body mass (kg)/stretch stature^2 (m), has been frequently used as the anthropometric indicator par excellence related to health. This index allows for a classification of the degree of obesity based on the values found in Table 9.1.

However, this index has shortcomings, especially in its use with infants and subjects with a large musculoskeletal development, as it is not able to differentiate components within body composition, so its analysis should be complemented with other indicators that allow understanding the subject's body composition.

Nevertheless, BMI is related to mortality and morbidity, being very low with values between 20 and 25; low between 25 and 30, moderate between 30 and 35; high between 35 and 40; and very high with values above 40.

The lowest risk of suffering from a coronary heart disease (CHD) is found with a BMI of 23, and each digit that increases the BMI above this value increases mortality from CHD by 2%. Thus, in subjects with a BMI above 30, compared to subjects with a BMI of 22.5–25, the prevalence of mortality increases by 30%, vascular pathology by 40%, diabetes by 60–120%, and neoplasia by 10%.

In addition, BMI has a significant and positive correlation with insulin resistance, gallbladder pathologies, systolic and diastolic blood pressure, and high cholesterol levels. However, BMI values below 20 are related to digestive and pulmonary pathologies.

9.4 Somatotype as a Health Indicator

The study of the somatotype in relation to health allows for the establishment of healthy somatozones. Thus, on the somatochart, we find a "health risk" zone located in the left/upper region of the Reuleaux triangle, where the value of the X axis is negative and the value of the Y axis is positive, while the healthiest patients have positive values on the X axis and negative values on the Y axis, being located further down and to the right on the somatochart.

In addition, previous research has shown that certain pathologies are related to endomorphy, mesomorphy, and ectomorphy, respectively. Thus, a higher endomorphy is related to endometrial cancer, cardiovascular diseases, obesity, diabetes, Down syndrome or dyslipidemias; a lower mesomorphy is related to cervical cancer, while a higher mesomorphy is related to cardiovascular disease, diabetes,

Down syndrome and dyslipidaemias; while a lower ectomorphy is related to Down syndrome.

9.5 Conicity Index as a Health Indicator

The conicity index (CI) allows for the analysis of abdominal fat mass by establishing a relationship between the waist girth, body mass and stretch stature. Thus, it quantifies the deviation of the girth of an imaginary cylinder, and the further it is from the unit (CI > 1) the more accumulation of fat mass it represents.

$$\text{Conicity index (CI)} = \frac{(\textit{Waist girth}\ (\text{cm})/10)}{0.109\sqrt{\frac{\textit{Body mass}\ (\text{kg})}{\textit{Stretch stature}\ (\text{cm})/10}}}$$

The conicity index itself has no units and its range oscillates between 1.00, which is the perfect cylinder, and 1.73, which is the perfect double cone. For example, if a person has a conicity index of 1.25, it means that this person has a waist girth that is 1.25 times larger than the girth of a cylinder that has been formed from the stretch stature and body mass of that person.

9.6 Analysis of Certain Pathologies Through Anthropometry

9.6.1 Anorexia Nervosa

In anorexia, there is a significant loss not only of fat mass, but also muscle mass. The percentage of fat mass described in anorexic patients is $7 \pm 2\%$, even being described below 5%. This pathology has a higher incidence in women.

9.6.2 Diabetes

Patients with insulin-dependent diabetes mellitus (IDDM), type 1, have a characteristic morphotype:

- Men: decreased waist/hip ratio and fat mass.
- Women: increased fat mass.

Therefore, patients with IDDM do not present a high body adiposity. However, glucose intolerance and non-insulin-dependent diabetes mellitus (NIDDM), also called type 2 diabetes, is related to the accumulation of abdominal subcutaneous fat mass.

The best prognostic factor for suffering from NIDDM is the antero-posterior abdominal breadth, with the highest quartiles having up to eleven times more probability of suffering from this disease. In addition, in type 2 diabetes, the waist girth, hips girth, and waist/hip ratio are considered very powerful prognostic factors for morbidity and mortality.

A proposal made by the International Diabetes Society lowers the healthy limits of waist girth to 80 cm for women and 94 cm for men.

9.6.3 Cardiovascular Pathology

In women, this pathology has a high correlation with larger waist girth, trunk skinfolds (subscapular, supraspinal and abdominal), subscapular/triceps ratio, waist/hip ratio, and endomorphy. Thus, previous research has shown that a waist/hip ratio greater than 0.85 in women may result in a significant increase in cardiac pathologies and comorbidities such as hypertension occurr.

In men, cardiovascular pathologies are associated with higher values in waist girth, BMI, waist/hip ratio, mesomorphy, and the "Y" axis of the somatochart. Similarly to women, when the waist/hip ratio in men exceeds 0.9–1, there is a significant increase in the presence of cardiac pathologies and comorbidities such as hypertension.

The etiopathogenesis of cardiovascular pathologies is related to the distribution of body adiposity. An excess of abdominal fat mass in men is associated with hypertension and ischemic heart disease.

Prognostic factors for cardiovascular morbidity and mortality in both sexes include skinfolds (especially the subscapular), waist girth, waist/hip ratio, and fat mass.

The skinfolds of the triceps and abdomen are directly proportional to cardiovascular risk, with protective levels being below 12 mm in men and 15 mm in women. Skinfolds with values higher than those indicated should be given special consideration. Specifically, the triceps skinfold has a significant relationship with hypertension, with a power similar to factors strongly involved in hypertensive pathology such as age, heart rate, alcohol intake, or family history of cardiovascular pathology.

9.6.4 Obesity

This is an epidemic problem, as considered by the World Health Organisation (WHO), which currently affects a large percentage of the world's population, mainly caused by changes in society's lifestyle.

Obesity is associated with hypertension, atherosclerosis, cardiovascular disease, congestive heart failure, type 2 diabetes, osteoarthritis, and some types of cancer, gallbladder, liver and kidney pathologies.

In addition, patients with metabolic syndrome (diabetes or glucose intolerance associated with dyslipidemia, obesity, and hypertension) have a larger waist girth, triceps skinfold, BMI, and mesomorphy, as well as lower ectomorphy values.

9.7 Conclusions from the Application of Anthropometry in the Health Field

To diagnose and monitor chronic pathologies based on anthropometry, the following can be used:

- Body mass index.
- Waist/hip ratio.
- Conicity index.
- Trunk skinfolds (triceps, subscapular, supraspinal and abdominal).

However, it is important to note that anthropometry is a non-invasive tool that complements medical examinations performed on patients to understand their health status.

9.8 Questionnaire

1. Anthropometry, with respect to health:
   (a) Has not demonstrated much usefulness scientifically.
   (b) Has been used for the prevention and monitoring of certain pathologies.
   (c) Cannot be used to control the effects of health-related interventions.
   (d) Is not useful for delving into the mechanisms of a pathology.
2. The two main utilities of anthropometry in the area of health area:
   (a) Treatment and prevention.
   (b) The identification of risk groups and treatment.
   (c) The prevention and identification of risk groups and the monitoring of the effects of treatments carried out in a population with a pathology.
   (d) None of the above.
3. How many measurements have shown the most relation with health?
   (a) 21, all from the restricted profile.
   (b) 18, nine from the restricted profile and nine from the complete profile.
   (c) 14, all from the complete profile.
   (d) 13, twelve from the restricted profile and one from the complete profile.
4. Regarding body mass:
   (a) The reduction of body mass can normalise blood pressure in hypertensive patients.
   (b) Body mass as an isolated variable is related to various pathologies.
   (c) Excessive and cyclical increases and decreases do not have implications for health.

   (d) All of the above are true.
5. Regarding skinfolds:
   (a) They can be used to locate the distribution of fat mass.
   (b) Skinfolds located on the trunk provide more information about health.
   (c) The ratio of subscapular/triceps skinfolds provides a representative value on the incidence of mortality in women.
   (d) All are true.
6. The waist/hip index is one of the most utilized in the health field, because:
   (a) It is very sensitive to changes in an individual's adiposity.
   (b) An increase in the value of this index indicates an increase in visceral fat mass.
   (c) It serves to know the relationship between muscle mass and adipose.
   (d) It is closely related to respiratory diseases.
7. The BMI has been frequently used for a long time. This index:
   (a) Allows for the classification of the degree of obesity of the patients.
   (b) Distinguishes well when overweightness is caused by an increase in muscle mass.
   (c) The lowest risk of suffering a coronary heart disease is found with a BMI above 23.
   (d) Only an excessively high BMI is related to certain pathologies.
8. Regarding the relationship of the somatotype and health, indicate the false one:
   (a) When the somatopoint is located in the upper left quadrant of the somatochart, there may be a health risk.
   (b) Values on the negative X axis and positive Y axis are related to patients who have good health.
   (c) Endomorphy has been associated with a higher risk of suffering from cardiovascular diseases.
   (d) Mesomorphy is related to a higher risk of suffering from cervical cancer.
9. The conicity index:
   (a) Relates the variables hips girth, body mass, and stretch stature.
   (b) Is an indicator of the accumulation of muscle mass.
   (c) If its value is greater than 1 it indicates accumulation of fat mass.
   (d) None of the above is true.
10. Regarding the analysis of certain pathologies through anthropometry:
   (a) Anorexia nervosa is characterised by high percentages of fat mass.
   (b) Type 2 diabetes mellitus is associated with accumulation of fat mass in the extremities.
   (c) The waist/hip ratio is not associated with cardiovascular pathology in either men or women.
   (d) All of the above are false.

Answers:
1.b 2.c 3.d 4.a 5.d 6.b 7.a 8.b 9.c 10.d

Bibliography

Boyko, E. J., Fujimoto, W. Y., Leonetti, D. L., & Newell-Morris, L. (2000). Visceral adiposity and risk of type 2 diabetes: A prospective study among Japanese Americans. *Diabetes Care, 23*(4), 465–471.

Caballero-García, M. F., Albaladejo-Saura, M., Vaquero-Cristóbal, R., & Esparza-Ros, F. (2022). Utility of the anthropometric variables in the diagnosis and characterisation of type 2 diabetes mellitus patients. *Journal of Sport and Health Research, 14*(3), 359–374.

Curilem Gatica, C., Almagià Flores, A., Yuing Farías, T., & Rodríguez Rodríguez, F. (2014). Body composition and heart rate variability in patients with chronic obstructive pulmonary disease pulmonary rehabilitation candidates. *Nutrición Hospitalaria, 30*(1), 179–182.

Expert Panel on the Identification, Evaluation, and Treatment of Overweight in Adults. (1998). Expert panel on the identification, evaluation, and treatment of overweight and obesity in adults. Executive summary of the clinical guidelines on the identification, evaluation, and treatment of overweight and obesity in adults. *International Archives of Internal Medicine, 158*(17), 1855–1867.

Marcos-Pardo, P. J., González-Gálvez, N., López-Vivancos, A., Espeso-García, A., Martínez-Aranda, L. M., Gea-García, G. M., Orquin-Castrillon, F. J., Carbonell-Baeza, A., Jimenez-Garcia, J. D., Velazquez-Diaz, D., Cadenas-Sanchez, C., Isidori, E., Fossati, C., Pigozzi, F., Rum, L., Norton, C., Tierney, A., Abelkalns, I., Klempere-Sipjagina, A., … Vaquero-Cristóbal, R. (2020). Sarcopenia, diet, physical activity and obesity in European middle-aged and older adults: The lifeage study. *Nutrients, 13*(1), 8.

Norton, K., & Olds, T. (1996). *Anthropometrica.* University of New South Wales Press.

Ross, R., Neeland, I. J., Yamashita, S., Shai, I., Seidell, J., Magni, P., Santos, R. D., Arsenault, B., Cuevas, A., Hu, F. B., Griffin, B. A., Zambon, A., Barter, P., Fruchart, J. C., Eckel, R. H., Matsuzawa, Y., & Després, J. P. (2020). Waist girth as a vital sign in clinical practice: A consensus statement from the IAS and ICCR working group on visceral obesity. *Nature Reviews Endocrinology, 16*(3), 177–189.

Sánchez Ferrer, M. (2011). *Study of the somatocarta in patients with chronic pathology.* Thesis. Miguel Hernández University.

Schorr, M., Dichtel, L. E., Gerweck, A. V., Valera, R. D., Torriani, M., Miller, K. K., & Bredella, M. A. (2018). Sex differences in body composition and association with cardiometabolic risk. *Biology of Sex Differences, 9*(1), 28.

Valdez, R., Seidell, J. C., Ahn, Y. I., & Weiss, K. M. (1993). A new index of abdominal adiposity as an indicator of risk for cardiovascular disease: A cross-population study. *International Journal of Obesity and Related Metabolic Disorders: Journal of the International Association for the Study of Obesity, 17*(2), 77–82.

Bibliography

FSC
www.fsc.org
MIX
Papier aus verantwortungsvollen Quellen
Paper from responsible sources
FSC® C105338

If you have any concerns about our products,
you can contact us on
ProductSafety@springernature.com

In case Publisher is established outside the EU,
the EU authorized representative is:
Springer Nature Customer Service Center GmbH
Europaplatz 3, 69115 Heidelberg, Germany

Printed by Libri Plureos GmbH
in Hamburg, Germany